Clinical Management of the Child and Teenager with Diabetes

THE JOHNS
HOPKINS PRESS
SERIES IN
AMBULATORY
PEDIATRIC
MEDICINE

Clinical Management of the Child and Teenager with Diabetes

LESLIE PLOTNICK, M.D.

Associate Professor of Pediatrics
Division of Pediatric Endocrinology
Director, Pediatric Diabetes
The Johns Hopkins University School of Medicine

and RANDI HENDERSON

Medical Writer

THE JOHNS HOPKINS UNIVERSITY PRESS
Baltimore & London

© 1998 The Johns Hopkins University Press
All rights reserved. Published 1998
Printed in the United States of America on acid-free paper
9 8 7 6 5 4 3 2 1

The Johns Hopkins University Press
2715 North Charles Street
Baltimore, Maryland 21218-4363
The Johns Hopkins Press Ltd., London
www.press.jhu.edu

Library of Congress Cataloging-in-Publication Data will be found at the end of this book.
A catalog record for this book is available from the British Library.

ISBN 0-8018-5908-5
ISBN 0-8018-5909-3 (pbk.)

Illustrations on pages 81 and 83 by Jacqueline Schaffer

Contents

Figures and Tables

FIGURES

TABLES

Preface

This is a tumultuous time in medicine. While science continues to provide new tools to treat disease, the framework for treatment is shifting. The traditional roles of primary care clinicians and specialists are being redefined. These are far-reaching changes that are transfiguring the face of medicine and patient care in America in the 1990s.

Within this context, the role of the primary care clinician in caring for children and adolescents with chronic diseases such as Type 1 diabetes (insulin-dependent diabetes mellitus) is rapidly changing. This comes at a time when the evidence for the importance of good control of diabetes has never been more clear and compelling. Patients whose diabetes is in good control have a better sense of physical and psychological well-being and a reduced risk of acute complications, including potentially life-threatening ketoacidosis. Also, in 1993, the results of a 10-year national study, the Diabetes Control and Complications Trial (DCCT), clearly showed that tighter blood glucose control could lower the risk of long-term complications, specifically retinopathy, nephropathy, and neuropathy.

A second factor is equally important. A growing body of research looks at possible "cures" for Type 1 diabetes. Some of these projects are exciting and may lead to at least a temporary "cure," perhaps in the next 10 to 20 years. The knowledge that a cure could happen in the lifetime of many patients, and the proof from the DCCT that control leads to fewer long-term complications, makes this a special time in history and increases clinicians' responsibility to help diabetes patients achieve the best control possible over their disease.

We are currently witnessing a shift from management of chronic disease by a specialty team to management by the primary care clinician. An important role will remain, however, for the specialty team. The best care will be provided when the primary care clinician establishes a productive and interactive working relationship with the specialty team and develops a thorough understanding of when diabetes management can come from the primary care provider and when consultation or referral is necessary. This book will provide guidelines for that, as well as a comprehensive patient management plan that can be applied to the individual needs of each patient.

Beginning in the 1970s and continuing through the 1980s, physicians treating children with Type 1 diabetes worked to develop specialty teams to address the multiple needs of their patients. This coincided in the late 1970s with the era of modern diabetes management. This era began with the availability of accurate home blood glucose monitoring and the measurement of glycosylated hemoglobin (also called glycohemoglobin, glycated hemoglobin, and HbA_{1C}). These advances enabled children with diabetes and their families to begin to take control of their diabetes and evaluate their status in a way that had never before been possible.

The specialty teams flourished in medical centers and large practices, fueled by the desire of practitioners to pair the technological advances that enabled home monitoring with the best information and education that they could provide to their patients. Specialty teams for Type 1 diabetes typically involve a nurse educator, a dietitian, a physician (who is usually an endocrinologist), and a mental health professional (who is usually a psychologist or clinical social worker).

An increasing realization of the burden of chronic pediatric disease and the complex educational needs of patients and their families highlighted the importance of the team approach. This approach is also used for the management of other chronic diseases in children, such as cystic fibrosis and gastrointestinal conditions such as Crohn's disease. There is no other condition, however, that demands as much home management as does diabetes.

The management routine for children with Type 1 diabetes can be emotionally draining and tremendously time-consuming. The work can seem never-ending. A wide constellation of factors in everyday life influence a child's blood glucose levels, and they change frequently—not even hourly, but from minute to minute. Stress, changes in routine, traveling, sleeping late, eating late, going to parties—these all affect blood glucose. The use of different types of insulin will produce different peaks and valleys in insulin levels. What's right on Monday may not be right on Tuesday. If a blood glucose level is too high, that is a problem; if it is too low, that is also a problem. A balance must constantly be maintained.

In addition, the consequences of wrong decisions or missed judgments may be threatening to health. Missing a dose of an antibiotic or a session of

Table 1.   **Sharing of Type 1 Diabetes Care Responsibilities between the Primary Care Clinician and the Specialty Team**

Primary Care Clinician Provides Type 1 Diabetes Care if	Specialty Team Provides Type 1 Diabetes Care if
Patient has satisfactory or good diabetes control (is meeting defined goals)	Patient is not meeting defined goals (has poor diabetes control)
Patient and family have low-intensity needs related to diabetes	Patient and family have high-intensity needs related to diabetes
Primary-care clinician has satisfactory skills, interest, and time for diabetes care	Primary-care clinician lacks skills, interest, or time for diabetes care

physical therapy usually poses little risk for a child with medical problems requiring these treatments. For the child with diabetes, missing a day of insulin is dangerous, as is receiving too much insulin.

Through the 1980s, specialty teams flowered and built a solid track record of competent and effective treatment, learning that nurses and dietitians were the key to helping patients and families manage Type 1 diabetes. One problem with this emphasis is that the role of primary care clinicians in chronic disease management tended to fade into the background. Fewer and fewer primary care clinicians felt comfortable managing Type 1 diabetes, and they deferred to the specialty teams.

This trend, of course, is now coming up against the changing face of medicine—the expanding presence of managed care and managed care's renewed emphasis on the role of the primary care clinician. There have been dramatic changes in recent years, with financial support for specialty teams diminishing and primary care clinicians expected increasingly to assume chronic disease management. This trend is likely to continue in the years to come.

There are several ways in which the specialty team and the primary care clinicians can work together, and it is likely that each practitioner will employ different systems for different patients, based on a number of factors (see table 1). These include the needs of the patient and family, the primary care clinician's skills and needs, the patient's level of comfort, the patient's success in meeting defined goals, the patient's managed care organization or insurance plan, and the geographic area.

A range of examples illustrates how such collaborations can work effectively:

> ➤ One example includes a full evaluation by the entire specialty team once a year, including HbA_{1C} measurement, update on research, com-

plication screening, and education and dietary update. If there are no issues impeding good control and the HbA_{1C} is in the target range, the primary care clinician will take over for the interval, with another full evaluation by the diabetes team scheduled in a year. If there are problems related to control—for example, if the family is not receiving the necessary education or the patient's glycohemoglobins are too high—then the team would see the patient more often.

➤ Alternatively, the primary care clinician might provide *all* Type 1 diabetes management or might refer the patient for specialty team consultation only as needed for a specific problem (i.e., poor blood glucose control) and provide all interim Type 1 diabetes management.

➤ In another scenario, the specialty team would see the patient every 3 months and do all Type 1 diabetes management, including management of day-to-day problems and sick days. This approach is usually most suitable to a large medical center where patients have relatively easy geographic access to the specialty team.

A customized combination of the above approaches will probably yield the best working relationship for most patients and their care providers. The best, most complete, and most flexible strategy for Type 1 diabetes management may be co-management or collaborative management, with the work being shared by the primary care clinician and specialty team, each of which would assume responsibility for specific aspects of helping a particular patient and family meet their goals. One general principle for primary care clinicians is that if goals are not being met, the patient should be referred for consultation. This is also applicable to the specialty team, who should consult with other specialists in the cases of patients who are difficult to manage and consistently have trouble meeting their goals.

The goal of this book is to provide the information that primary care clinicians need to treat children and adolescents with Type 1 diabetes. This includes an understanding of the family issues that are involved, because family involvement is an integral part of diabetes management for children. Information about the specific services provided by each member of the specialty team will be presented in a way that will be useful and valuable for primary care clinicians, and day-to-day issues of management as well as acute situations will be addressed.

How to Use This Book

This is a practical how-to book, and we have attempted to present the information in as useful a form as possible. The many aspects of Type 1 diabetes care are interrelated. You will note that the message about the importance of good control and the descriptions of methods to achieve it are repeated throughout the book—however, different considerations are emphasized in different chapters. *To make it easier for the clinician to focus on the skills and medical tasks required for the child or teenager being treated, we have organized the content around various points in the diabetes spectrum of care and the age of the child.* This approach also leads to some repetition, although the reader is asked in some instances to refer to other chapters for more detailed explanations of concepts and techniques.

A few notes about style: First, equal numbers of girls and boys develop Type 1 diabetes. We have tried to balance the use of feminine and masculine pronouns, alternating them throughout the text. Second, when we speak of clinicians, we are speaking of the variety of health care providers who interact with children and teenagers with diabetes and their families. This includes—but is not necessarily limited to—pediatricians, internists, family physicians, nurse practitioners, nurse educators, physician assistants, dietitians and nutritionists, and mental health counselors. When we use the term *clinician*, we are referring to anyone who is providing the care in the circumstances being discussed, and we usually do not specify whether we are referring to a primary care clinician or specialist, or to a nurse or physician, since care may be rendered by either one or both. In the following pages, *we* refers to members of the Johns Hopkins pediatric diabetes team or, more generally, to clinicians treating children with diabetes.

Acknowledgments

We wish to thank the following people, without whom this book would not have been possible: Jackie Wehmueller, our editor at the Johns Hopkins University Press, whose support and encouragement since the inception of this project are deeply appreciated; Loretta Clark, RN, CDE, for painstakingly reviewing our manuscript, and for her expertise in caring for patients and their families; Richard Rubin, Ph.D., CDE—on whose principles the chapter on psychological issues is based—for his contributions to the Johns Hopkins diabetes program; our families, for their understanding and continuing support during our work on this project; and children and adolescents with diabetes and their families, from whom all our real knowledge comes and who are an ongoing source of inspiration. We owe special thanks to the individuals who participated in the discussion in chapter 12.

In addition, we appreciate the input from Christopher Saudek, M.D.; Lauren Bogue, M.D.; and Carol Parnes, M.D., and Michael May, M.D., and their office staff.

Clinical Management of the Child and Teenager with Diabetes

Introduction

Twenty-five years ago, when I (L.P.) began treating children with diabetes, we were dealing with imperfect gauges and uncertain management. Monitoring was based on urine testing. The children would dip their urine three or four times a day to check for glucose or ketones. Glucose measures ranged from negative to 5 percent, ketones went from negative to large, and that was all that patients could ascertain. No highs, no lows. Patients had no way of measuring hypoglycemia, except by symptoms. To get a blood glucose level, the blood had to be sent to a laboratory, and sometimes it took hours to get results.

By today's standards, management was very loose. Most patients took one or two insulin shots per day, but it was very hard to judge what doses to give. With no glycohemoglobin measure, we had no precise idea what the patient's level of control was. We really were shooting in the dark. In some sense, management was easier, because with fewer known variables to factor in, there was simply less to do. All that was required of patients was that they watch their diets, eat the same amount at the same time every day, avoid simple sugars, take their insulin shots, and check their urine several times a day. Many people hated checking urine and didn't even do that. Insulin came in two different strengths—U-40 and U-80—each of which had its own size syringe, leaving room for the error of using the wrong syringe and injecting half or double the intended dose. In addition, insulin was not as highly purified as it is today, leading to more frequent skin lipoatrophy or hypertrophy from the injections.

With modern management, patients have better diabetes control and fewer complications. We can't tell patients that if they keep good control, they have no risk of complications, just as we can't tell someone that if he is a good driver he has no risk of being in a traffic accident. But the results that are now available and are still emerging from ongoing clinical trials make it clear that our intuitive feelings that better diabetes control means better quality of life (and perhaps longer life) are scientifically valid.

I became a pediatrician because I liked the fact that in pediatrics I could offer an intervention that could substantially change someone's life. As a pediatrician I was drawn to the subspecialty of endocrinology because the endocrine hormones are so critical to so many aspects of human life and development, and the medications in endocrinology are often replacements for normal body hormones.

I was also attracted to the psychological and behavioral aspects of endocrine problems. In pediatric endocrinology, one must consider the whole child in the whole family. The chronicity of most endocrine conditions ensures ongoing contact with the patient and family. Clinicians become part of the lives of these families. Many of our children, particularly diabetes patients, "age out" of our practice after we have followed them through childhood and adolescence.

The children we treated in the early 1970s went through the revolutionizing of diabetes care through home blood glucose monitoring and glycohemoglobin measurement. More than ever, these changes emphasized the family context of care. Home monitoring shifted the responsibility of diabetes management from the health care provider to the family. There are many variables that affect blood glucose, and there are many variables that affect an individual's ability to live with diabetes. These are best known and best understood by the individual and the family. Health care providers may know diabetes better, but we can never know the child better. We must think of the family as the primary caregivers, and the health care providers as consultants.

Families, then, need to be active participants in their child's care, and they must be willing to learn what they need to know to do this. Education of patients and families is one of the most critical components of diabetes treatment, the link that makes family management possible. It is the responsibility of health care providers to help families understand their role in management and to furnish information and supporting materials that will tell them what they need to know, both the basics and the nuances.

Clinicians working with children with diabetes and their families must have comprehensive knowledge and the ability to teach. They must enjoy explaining things and be willing to go over them again and again. There must be mutual trust between the family and the clinician, and it is the role of the clinician to foster this trust, to assure the family that we are working with them to achieve common goals.

It is also important to understand that knowledge does not equal behavior. In addition to learning the skills to perform the necessary technical tasks and the cognitive ability to make management decisions, many families need to learn to improve the behaviors that are important to successful diabetes management.

Records are the best tools for learning and can be reviewed at family meetings and meetings with the health care provider. Without written records, your problem-solving ability is limited. When things are not going well, you want more information, more complete recordkeeping. This will allow for early action at the beginning of a problem, to help prevent the situation from getting out of control. The better the control, the more normal the life of the child and family with diabetes can be.

Parents, siblings, and the child or teen with diabetes must learn how to make management decisions within certain limits that are established in collaboration with the clinician. They must understand that diabetes is a 24-hour-a-day, 7-day-a-week condition. They need to learn how to recognize early signs and symptoms of trouble and know when to call for consultation. Only the family can make minute-to-minute, hour-to-hour interventions, observing when something is beginning to get out of control, and taking quick corrective action. As problems occur, families and health care providers must solve problems together and learn from the problems and solutions.

Over time, as the family becomes increasingly confident and competent, the role of the health care provider diminishes. The goal is to have the child and family in charge, not the diabetes. The alternative is to let diabetes overshadow all facets of their lives, with the result that the child is not healthy enough to live a normal life and moves from one crisis to another with a less than hopeful long-term prognosis.

Diabetes is forever, an inescapable fact that can be very discouraging to some people. Much of what health care providers can do, especially for families just beginning to deal with the diabetes diagnosis, is to keep hope alive. The best service we can provide is to help families cope and to help them stay interested in self-management. Nearly all children and teenagers with diabetes, as well as their families, have the desire and the ability to learn how to manage their disease. Health care providers—specialists, nurses, primary care physicians, dietitians, and social workers—may sometimes underestimate this desire and ability.

There are a number of institutions and resources that can help with these tasks. We recommend that families join the American Diabetes Association and the Juvenile Diabetes Foundation, and that younger children consider attending diabetes camps. Almost every state has such a camp, and financial assistance is often available for needy families. Older children can consider working as counselors at diabetes camps.

Much of the discussion in the following pages will examine problems encountered by patients and their families. You will meet children and teenagers with diabetes and see how they manage their disease with varying degrees of success. A sketch of Amy M., a girl whom we began treating when she was 6 years old, will help to set an encouraging and optimistic tone. Amy has taught us all some lessons about how to cope with this demanding disease. She is one of many children who manage diabetes intelligently and competently in a way that allows them to lead full lives with minimal restrictions.

CASE STUDY.   Amy M. was diagnosed when she was 6 years old. She had polyuria and polydypsia of 2 weeks' duration, but no other symptoms and no weight loss. Her height was 115.1 centimeters (45.3 in.), in the 50th percentile for her age; her weight was 21.0 kilograms (46.2 lb), in the 75th percentile. Her urine was positive for glucose and ketones, and her blood glucose was 263 milligrams per deciliter (mg/dL). Her pediatrician diagnosed Type 1 diabetes.

Amy is an only child; her father is a teacher, and her mother is a nurse who works part-time. Amy's initial insulin doses were 4 units of NPH and 3 of Regular in the morning and 3 units of NPH and 1 of Regular at dinner. (See chapter 6 for a description of insulin types.) From the start, she demonstrated excellent blood glucose control. Her insulin dosage was gradually adjusted to maintain optimal control and correlate with her growth. Her linear growth was normal, with her height remaining between the 50th and 75th percentile and her weight in the 75th percentile.

Three years after diagnosis, Amy's glycohemoglobin counts remained in the target range most of the time, reflecting consistent control. She was supervised regularly by her parents, and they are very effective problem-solvers together.

When she was 10$^{1}/_{2}$, Amy started on an insulin pump, at her own and her family's request. She wanted the pump in order to ensure good control. Amy's meal plan is set so that she consumes about 70 grams of carbohydrate at each meal and 40 grams at each snack, and she determines her insulin doses on the basis of carbohydrate consumption (1 unit for every 10 to 15 g of carbohydrates), with a sliding scale based on her body weight (then 35 kg) that goes up or down a half unit for every 25 mg/dL of blood glucose outside her target range. She uses two basal rates, one from 10 A.M. to 3 A.M., and a slightly higher one from 3 A.M. to 10 A.M.

Amy enjoyed both the freedom and the enhanced control that the pump provided, but she initially had a problem inserting the pump catheter, which must be changed a few times a week. She found the procedure very painful but began using a topical anesthetic, which she applied about an hour before inserting the catheter. Once the problem of pain was solved, Amy did very well on the pump.

Amy is now 14, 163 centimeters (64 in.) tall and weighing 59 kilograms (130 lb); her height and weight are both in the 75th percentile for her age. She has adult sexual maturation. Her glycemic control is very good, although there are intervals when it is less than ideal. She monitors her blood glucose three to five times a day, so that she can make insulin dose adjustments when necessary. Her glycohemoglobin readings are consistently in target range, and her glycohemoglobin was 6.0 percent (of total hemoglobin) at her last visit (normal: 4.5 to 6.1%). Her blood glucose is generally in the normal range, between 70 and 120 mg/dL, and there are no signs of any complications.

While these facts and figures of diabetes are a routine part of her everyday life, Amy's life goes much beyond diabetes. She gets A's and B's in school, plays on the girls' basketball team, loves rock music, and—like many girls her age—records her thoughts and feelings in a diary.

1

Overview

Type 1 diabetes (or insulin-dependent diabetes mellitus) is a complex and multifaceted disease that has an impact on numerous and varied aspects of the lives of patients and their families. The diagnosis of Type 1 diabetes is usually straightforward, and its presentation is typically dramatic and rarely subtle. Management of Type 1 diabetes is a major long-term challenge for the child, the family, and the health care providers. It involves consideration of complex medical, psychological, behavioral, and educational issues. There are few—if any—other diseases that require the intensity of self-management that Type 1 diabetes demands.

The central and immediate cause of Type 1 diabetes is insulin deficiency. The underlying causes of the destruction of the insulin-producing beta cells in the pancreatic islets are becoming increasingly better understood and will be reviewed below. Because of insulin deficiency, patients with the disease need exogenous insulin for survival. Replacement of insulin with currently available methods is *not* truly physiologic, even with newer techniques. It is an imperfect system. Insulin requirements vary, and subcutaneous insulin injections do not truly mimic the finely tuned process of normal pancreatic insulin secretion.

From these points—the requirement for insulin replacement and the imperfection of existing methods of insulin delivery—come all the management issues and problems and the risk of acute and long-term complications which comprise the subject matter of this book.

This chapter reviews the pathophysiology, diagnostic criteria, etiology, genetics and natural history, epidemiology and statistics, and clinical course of Type 1 diabetes.

DEFINITION AND DIAGNOSIS

Diabetes is currently classified into two main categories, which encompass the vast majority of people with diabetes. A new classification system was developed and published in 1997 (*Diabetes Care*, suppl. 1, 21:S5–19, 1998).

Type 1 diabetes is due to beta cell damage resulting in absolute insulin deficiency. Patients with the disorder are prone to ketoacidosis, and death will occur without insulin treatment. This category includes the majority of patients in whom beta cell destruction is due to autoimmunity, as well as those few whose diabetes has an unknown cause (i.e., is idiopathic).

Type 1 diabetes was previously called insulin-dependent diabetes mellitus (IDDM), juvenile-onset diabetes mellitus (JODM), or ketosis-prone diabetes mellitus. Patients may be of any age but are usually children or adolescents when diagnosed. A small minority of patients with Type 1 diabetes have no evidence of autoimmunity.

Type 2 diabetes is the more prevalent form. This type of diabetes is due primarily to insulin resistance, with inadequate insulin secretion to compensate for this resistance; that is, it indicates a relative, not an absolute, insulin deficiency. It was previously called non-insulin-dependent diabetes mellitus (NIDDM), or adult-onset diabetes (AODM).

Most patients who have Type 2 diabetes are obese, with an increased amount of abdominal fat. Weight reduction may produce a decrease in insulin resistance, and oral agents are often successful for treatment. Type 2 diabetes has a strong genetic association, and its risk rises with age, body weight, and physical inactivity. Although patients with Type 2 diabetes do not require insulin therapy for survival, they may need it for treatment of hyperglycemia.

Other specific types of diabetes also occur. These are due to causes such as genetic defects of the beta cell, genetic defects in insulin action, and diseases of the exocrine pancreas (including cystic fibrosis).

When genetic abnormalities in beta cell function produce diabetes, the resulting forms usually cause mild hyperglycemia at an early age, are inherited in an autosomal dominant fashion, and cause impaired insulin secretion with minimal or no problems in insulin sensitivity. Some of these forms are due to specific, identified mutations, one of which produces a defect in glucokinase. Diabetes in this category has been called maturity onset diabetes of youth (MODY).

Sometimes it is unclear whether patients have Type 1 or Type 2 diabetes, and in such cases further evaluation and careful follow-up may be needed. Although this book focuses on Type 1 diabetes, many of the principles discussed here also apply to patients with Type 2 diabetes, particularly those who take insulin.

The diagnosis of Type 1 diabetes is straightforward and rarely subtle. Children and adolescents who have the classic symptoms—polyuria, polyphagia, polydipsia, weight loss, and fatigue—and have a random blood glucose greater than 200 mg/dL with glycosuria and often ketonuria (with or without ketonemia and acidosis) clearly have diabetes.

The new classification system indicates three ways to diagnosis diabetes and states that (in the absence of unequivocal hyperglycemia and metabolic decompensation) the diagnosis must be confirmed on a subsequent day by one of the three following criteria:

1. symptoms, in combination with a random (casual, or any-time-of-day) plasma glucose equal to or greater than 200 mg/dL;
2. fasting plasma glucose equal to or greater than 126 mg/dL (after at least 8 hr with no caloric intake);
3. an oral glucose tolerance test (OGTT) of 1.75 grams of glucose per kilogram of body weight (maximum glucose: 75 g) with the 2-hour level equal to or greater than 200 mg/dL.

Other test results are defined as follows:

1. fasting plasma glucose less than 110 mg/dL—normal;
2. fasting plasma glucose equal to or greater than 110 mg/dL and less than 126—impaired fasting glucose;

3. fasting plasma glucose equal to or greater than 126 mg/dL—diabetes; requires confirmation.

OGTT results (given as plasma glucose levels) are defined as follows:

1. less than 140 mg/dL 2 hours after oral glucose—normal;
2. 140 to 199 mg/dL 2 hours after oral glucose—impaired glucose tolerance;
3. 200 mg/dL or greater 2 hours after oral glucose—diabetes; requires confirmation.

Oral glucose tolerance tests are rarely necessary for the diagnosis of Type 1 diabetes in children and adolescents.

Not all children and adolescents with high blood glucose (greater than 200 mg/dL) have Type 1 diabetes. In some individuals, high blood glucose levels can be secondary to certain medications and hormonal excesses; this is most commonly seen in cases of treatment with pharmacologic doses of glucocorticoids for underlying diseases (e.g., autoimmune diseases, leukemia, reactive airway disease, kidney disease, inflammatory bowel disease). Even though these individuals do not have beta cell destruction, they still need insulin to treat the hyperglycemia while they remain on steroids. Because glucocorticoid therapy (and the rare hormonal excess syndromes such as pheochromocytoma, Cushing's syndrome, pituitary gigantism, and acromegaly) produce insulin resistance, higher doses of insulin than are used for Type 1 diabetes are usually needed to control hyperglycemia in patients with these disorders.

Children with cystic fibrosis may also develop diabetes. This is due in part to fibrosis, fatty infiltration, and disruption of the normal internal structure of the pancreas which contributes to islet destruction.

ETIOLOGY AND GENETICS

Type 1 diabetes is an autoimmune disease. In the past two decades, our understandings of immunology in general, and the process of beta cell destruction specifically, have increased tremendously. These understandings have great significance and may eventually lead to prevention and cure of diabetes.

Table 1.1.   **Risk of an Individual Developing Type 1 Diabetes if a Sibling Has the Disease**

Relationship	Risk (%)
Identical twins	≤50
HLA identical	15–20
HLA haploidentical	5
HLA nonidentical	≤1

There is no single diabetes gene. Most likely there is a series of unfortunate genetic combinations or alterations that increase the risk of beta cell damage. Human lymphocyte antigens (HLA) DR3 and DR4 seem to play an important role and convey an increased risk; one or both of these antigens are present in about 95 percent of all people with Type 1 diabetes. A person who inherits either DR3 or DR4 has a 3- to 5-fold increased risk of developing Type 1 diabetes, while inheritance of *both* DR3 and DR4 confers a 10- to 20-fold risk. DQ antigen variations may also account for changes in the risk of developing Type 1 diabetes. For example, an amino acid variation at position 57 on the DQ beta chain, non-aspartic acid, is associated with a significant increase in risk. In addition to HLA, other genes on different chromosomes may also be implicated in susceptibility to Type 1 diabetes. There are also indications that certain other genetic alterations raise or lower the risk of beta cell damage.

However, the pattern of development of Type 1 diabetes in identical twins makes it clear that it is most likely a *susceptibility* to the disease that is inherited, rather than the disease itself. When one identical twin has Type 1 diabetes, the other twin develops the disease half the time or less. This inherited susceptibility appears to place the beta cell at unusual risk for immunologic inflammatory damage. (Specific autoantibodies are reviewed in the next section.) The importance of external environmental factors in the process of beta cell damage is supported by this 50 percent or less concordance of Type 1 diabetes in identical twins, as well as by the marked geographic variation in incidence.

The risk of an individual developing Type 1 diabetes if one sibling has the disease is shown in table 1.1. Overall, approximately 5 percent of siblings of people with Type 1 diabetes will also develop Type 1 diabetes.

While Type 1 diabetes symptoms usually emerge suddenly, the process of beta cell destruction appears to take place over months to years. It is immune-mediated. There is some controversy over whether this is a relentless, progressive process that will inevitably produce Type 1 diabetes or whether the process may wax and wane over time and sometimes enter remission. The external environmental factors associated with this process may involve either recurrent and intermittent exposure or continuous exposure but are unlikely to occur in the form of a single triggering event. Environmental factors include viruses, toxins, specific foods, and possibly stress.

Cytokines released by the autoimmune process destroy the beta cells, either directly or by generating oxygen free radicals. (Beta cells have low levels of antioxidants.) There are likely to be two phases in the process of beta cell destruction: an early, cytokine-dependent initiation phase and a later phase with antigen-specific T-lymphocyte proliferation that amplifies and perpetuates beta cell destruction. Beta cell protective mechanisms such as enzymes that protect against the damage caused by free radicals can help beta cells resist immunologic damage.

It appears, then, that susceptibility to Type 1 diabetes is conferred by unfavorable combinations of beta cell–destructive and beta cell–protective mechanisms and common gene alleles for HLA. Specific HLA types appear to be necessary for the development of Type 1 diabetes but are not sufficient on their own to cause disease unless they are augmented by external environmental factors.

PATHOPHYSIOLOGY

Without insulin, the body loses its ability to utilize its fuel. Glucose, the body's main energy source, is no longer metabolized but builds up in the blood and passes through in the urine. The word *diabetes* is from the Greek for "siphon," or "pass through."

Insulin is the major anabolic hormone produced by the body. When food is ingested, insulin stimulates energy storage in the forms of glycogen, protein, and fat tissue. When insulin levels are low or deficient, the tissue uptake of glucose is inhibited and stored energy substrate is mobilized (glycogenolysis, proteolysis, and lipolysis). Since insulin is a potent antilipolytic hormone, a greater degree of insulin deficiency is required for lipolysis (breakdown of fat stores) to occur than for hyperglycemia to occur. Therefore, in the early stages of insulin deficiency, hyperglycemia is the primary feature. As a more severe degree of insulin deficiency develops, ketonuria, ketonemia, and acidosis may occur.

For diabetic ketoacidosis (DKA) to occur, there must be not only insulin deficiency but also a relative excess of counterregulatory hormones (glucagon, catecholamines, growth hormone, and cortisol). Hyperglycemia leads to an osmotic diuresis, causing the symptoms of polyuria and polydipsia. Passive electrolyte loss occurs along with the osmotic diuresis. Weight loss ensues because of the general catabolic state, as well as the osmotic diuresis. Eventually, dehydration results. If the child cannot drink enough fluid to compensate for the diuresis, as in the case of vomiting or decreased level of consciousness, dehydration will be particularly severe. Lipolysis results in ketone production, which causes a metabolic acidosis.

This information leads to several important practical points:

> Insulin deficiency is not only a disease of glucose regulation. It also affects protein and fat metabolism.
> People with insulin deficiency need exogenous insulin to prevent lipolysis and proteolysis. It is needed both to cover the calories from eating (to prevent elevated blood glucose and to move the glucose into the cells for energy) and to turn off excess production of glucose from internal sources (primarily the liver). This is why insulin must be given not only to cover food intake but also during periods of fasting (e.g., overnight or when illness or other factors make eating impossible for longer periods).
> Ketones indicate that lipolysis is occurring, a sign of relative or absolute insulin deficiency.

NATURAL HISTORY

The natural history of the beta cell defect (or of Type 1 diabetes) appears to have several stages that most often occur over a period of years but may occasionally be completed within months (fig. 1.1). There is, first, an underlying genetic predisposition or susceptibility based on an individual's genes, as discussed in the previous section. Then a trigger (or triggers) occurs, initiating an autoimmune process.

The timing and nature of these triggers are still unknown. Most theories look at certain environmental factors that can induce this autoimmunity; these include viruses, toxins, specific foods, and possibly stress. One controversial theory is that cow's milk introduced to infants may, by a process of "molecular mimicry," induce antibodies to a specific beta cell antigen. This process may involve humoral and/or cell-mediated autoimmune

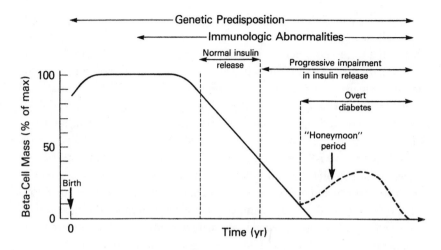

Fig. 1.1. Natural history of beta cell defect. Timing of trigger in relation to immunologic abnormalities is unknown. Note that overt diabetes is not apparent until insulin secretory reserves are < 10 to 20 percent of normal.
American Diabetes Association, Medical Management of Insulin-Dependent (Type I) Diabetes, *2d ed. (Alexandria, Va.: ADA, 1994).*

phenomena and is identified by measurement of specific autoantibodies: islet cell antibodies (ICAs), insulin autoantibodies (IAAs), and antiglutamic acid decarboxylase (anti-GAD) antibodies.

Early in this process, there is measurable evidence of the autoimmune process but there are no detectable metabolic abnormalities. As the autoimmune process progresses, the first metabolic abnormality that can be detected is a decrease in the first-phase (initial) insulin response to intravenous (IV) glucose on an IV glucose tolerance test. With further decrease in beta cell mass and insulin secretory capacity, blood glucose elevations occur after oral glucose (or caloric intake); later, increased blood glucose occurs even if the patient is fasting. Finally, overt Type 1 diabetes is manifested. Most (80% to 90%) of the beta cell mass must be lost before overt Type 1 diabetes occurs.

Thus, while the onset of Type 1 diabetes often seems acute, particularly when it coincides with a recent viral illness, the underlying autoimmune destructive process has been occurring over a long period, probably years.

Attempts to use immunosuppression in newly diagnosed Type 1 diabetes patients have produced short-term remissions. Therefore, new ideas include the theory that immunosuppression or intervention should be started earlier in the process of beta cell destruction, when there is greater beta cell mass and therefore more insulin secretory capacity. It is hoped that in the future clinicians will be able to *prevent* Type 1 diabetes by intervening earlier in the autoimmune process. This possibility is currently under investigation in the Diabetes Prevention Trial (DPT-1), a national study sponsored by the National Institutes of Health. The DPT-1 is attempting to screen approximately 80,000 individuals under the age of 45 who are first-degree relatives of people with Type 1 diabetes. Those subjects with positive islet cell antibodies, positive insulin autoantibodies, and a decreased first-phase insulin release in an IV glucose tolerance test will be given several preventive therapies. This trial is initially using subcutaneous insulin for high-risk relatives and oral insulin for moderate-risk relatives. Eventually, purified glutamic acid decarboxylase (or another antigen) may be used in another oral trial. These are initial attempts to induce immunologic tolerance to specific beta cell antigens in the hope that this will prevent further beta cell damage and therefore prevent Type 1 diabetes.

The hope is that such a trial can identify those individuals with positive immune markers who seem destined to develop Type 1 diabetes within a few years. Even if these people need to take two shots of insulin a day for life to maintain significant beta cell function and metabolic normalcy with normal glycohemoglobin levels, such a prophylactic regimen may enable them to avoid all of the long-term complications of Type 1 diabetes and most of the short-term ones (except for occasional hypoglycemic episodes). This would be a major success in treatment and would improve the quality of life of the person with Type 1 diabetes—even if it is not a total cure.

EPIDEMIOLOGY AND STATISTICS

In 1995, according to the National Diabetes Information Clearinghouse (*Diabetes in America*, 2d ed., NIH Publication no. 95-1468 [n.p.: NIDDK, 1995]), there were an estimated 8 million diagnosed cases of diabetes in the United States. The vast majority of these were Type 2, or noninsulin dependent. (Another estimated 8 million cases of Type 2 diabetes are undiagnosed.) The estimated number of Type 1 diabetes cases is about 800,000, with 100,000 to 127,000 occurring in children or adolescents under the age of 19. There are about 30,000 new cases of Type 1 diabetes diagnosed each year in the United States.

Type 1 diabetes in children and adolescents is more prevalent than other severe chronic pediatric diseases, such as cancer, cystic fibrosis, sickle cell disease, and juvenile rheumatoid arthritis. Prevalence studies of Type 1 diabetes in the United States vary, but most indicate a prevalence of 1.2 to 1.9 per 1,000 population. Incidence (the number of new cases per year per 100,000 population) is a more accurate statistic. Worldwide, the incidence of the disease ranges from less than 1 per 100,000 to 35 per 100,000, depending on geographic area. The United States has an intermediate incidence of 8 to 18 per 100,000, with a mean of about 15. Interestingly, the incidence of Type 1 diabetes has a statistically significant positive correlation with the distance of the specific country from the equator: the farther from the equator, the higher the incidence of Type 1 diabetes. The same association is shown by an inverse correlation of the incidence of Type 1 diabetes with the mean annual temperature. The lower the temperature, the higher the incidence of Type 1 diabetes. These associations support the importance of both genetic predispositions and environmental influences and triggers in the development of Type 1 diabetes.

The incidence of Type 1 diabetes increases with age in the pediatric age group. Type 1 diabetes is rare in infants and toddlers. After age 2, the incidence increases steadily until it peaks in adolescence; it then declines in the late teens. The peak incidence in girls is more than 18 months earlier than the peak incidence in boys, consistent with the earlier onset of puberty in girls. Overall, the incidence rates in males and females are approximately equal.

An interesting observation is that new cases of Type 1 diabetes have a seasonal distribution, with more cases diagnosed in the colder winter months than in the summer. The reasons for this distribution are unclear, but it is observed in all geographic areas.

Even though Type 1 diabetes is a relatively common disease, the meaning of the prevalence rates to the individual child is that an elementary-school child in a moderate-sized school will often be the only one in the school with diabetes. In a large high school (one with more than 1,000 students), there will often be only 2 or 3 students with diabetes. It is easy to understand why it is not unusual for the child with diabetes to feel alone and isolated, and to know no other children with diabetes.

COSTS OF DIABETES

The costs related to Type 1 diabetes care are considerable. In the United States in 1992, the direct medical costs attributed to diabetes approximated $45 billion. An additional $47 billion in indirect costs (i.e., disability, work loss, and premature mortality) emphasize what an expensive disease this is.

In the Diabetes Control and Complications Trial, the annual costs per patient per year were compared in the categories of conventional care (one to two blood glucose tests and one to two insulin injections per day), intensive treatment with multiple daily injections (more than four shots daily), and continuous subcutaneous insulin infusion (insulin pumps). The findings were

> ➤ about $1,700 per patient per year for conventional care;
> ➤ $4,000 per patient per year for multiple daily injections; and
> ➤ $5,800 per patient per year for an insulin pump.

The major differences are due to the number of outpatient visits, the costs of blood glucose self-monitoring supplies, and the costs of pump supplies. Intensive management costs 2 to 3 times as much as conventional care, and pumps cost 1.5 times as much as multiple daily injections.

One way of evaluating these costs is by comparing them to the costs of diabetes complications. The long-term complications of Type 1 diabetes, which are reviewed in detail in chapter 10, include a number of chronic—and costly—conditions. For example, the cost per patient per year is approximately $2,000 for blindness and $45,000 for end-stage renal disease (ESRD); the cost is nearly $30,000 per patient per event for lower-extremity amputation. And these costs do not include the "cost" of human suffering.

The DCCT intensive treatment regimen will lead to improved quality of life; a net increase in years of good vision, years without ESRD, and years without lower extremity amputations; and some gain in length of life. Analyses of the benefits of the DCCT intensive treatment regimen found the delayed time to first complications to be about 15 years and projected the prolongation of life to be greater than 5 years. Therefore, it seems clear that intensive treatment of Type 1 diabetes is cost-effective, although it may not be cost-saving (W. H. Herman et al., "The Cost-Effectiveness of Intensive Insulin Therapy for Diabetes Mellitus," *Endocrinology and Metabolism Clinics of North America* 26:679–95, 1997). Specific costs of supplies are listed in Appendix A.

Medical Presentation and Initial Management

MEDICAL PRESENTATION

Patients with Type 1 diabetes present with a spectrum of symptoms, ranging from mild to severe. The severity of these symptoms depends upon the degree of insulin deficiency—that is, how much or how little insulin the body is continuing to produce. In a person with a very mild insulin deficiency, the first manifestation of the condition might be higher than normal blood glucose after meals, but no remarkable symptoms.

While the condition can go unnoticed at this point, it is not uncommon for a clinician to see this presentation. Children often come for a checkup after school and an afterschool snack, turning up a routine urinalysis that is positive for glucose. This can lead to a diagnosis of diabetes even though there have been no apparent symptoms, although upon questioning it may be disclosed that there has been an increase in urinary frequency, lack of weight gain, or some weight loss.

At the other extreme of the spectrum is a child

whose early symptoms were missed or misdiagnosed and who may suddenly become extremely ill with ketoacidosis. In such a case, the symptoms often include lethargy and vomiting. If not treated promptly, the child will become increasingly acidotic, dehydrated, and unarousable.

For primary care clinicians, it will be helpful to recognize various different presentations of Type 1 diabetes. The following four cases illustrate the variety of ways in which this disease can first be manifested and observed. The first two cases were detected later than they should have been. Symptoms were missed or not attended to by parents or the health care provider. In contrast, Emily and Bobby, the third and fourth patients described, were picked up early because of attentive parents or health care providers.

CASE STUDY.   Kristen D., aged 2 years, was originally brought by her parents to her pediatrician because of concerns about lack of energy and loss of weight. According to family measurements, Kristen had lost 5 pounds in 2 weeks, from a weight of about 31 pounds. Her parents also reported about 2 days of polyuria and polydipsia.

The pediatrician was unable to obtain a urine sample (which is not unusual in a child this age) and sent Kristen home. He did not take blood to check for glucose or ask the family to bring in a urine sample. At home Kristen's symptoms worsened, and she began to have deep, rapid respirations. Her parents again brought her to the pediatrician, who diagnosed reactive airway disease (asthma), administered albuterol nebulization in the office, and sent her home with albuterol syrup. The symptoms worsened at home, with Kristen's breathing becoming more labored, and her parents brought her to the emergency department of a local hospital. In the emergency department, Kussmaul respirations (the labored breathing that is characteristic of acidosis) were noted. Kristen was dehydrated and poorly arousable. Her initial pH was 6.9, her blood glucose was 868 mg/dL, and her serum bicarbonate was 2 milliequivalents per liter (mEq/L). She was diagnosed with Type 1 diabetes, given intravenous fluids and insulin in the emergency department, and admitted to the pediatric intensive care unit, where she remained for 36 hours.

CASE STUDY.   Susan M. was 13½ years old when, over a period of 6 weeks, her parents noticed that she was feeling increasingly fatigued, with headaches and dizziness. They thought that she sometimes seemed dazed and "out of it" and asked her if she was taking drugs. Susan denied any drug use. Her parents accepted her answer and did not seek medical attention despite intensifying symptoms, which included polyuria and polydipsia, and then nausea and vomiting. After about a week of nausea, Susan's parents took her to a community health center with vomiting, dizziness, and some chest pain. She also appeared to have poor peripheral perfusion, and her urine was positive for glucose and ketones. Susan was sent to the emergency department, where her pH was 6.95 and her blood glucose was 459 mg/dL. She was diagnosed with Type 1 diabetes and admitted to the pediatric intensive care unit.

CASE STUDY.   Emily G. was 12 years old, a healthy child seeing her pediatrician for a routine checkup. Her height was 146 centimeters (4 ft, 9.5 in.), in the 25th percentile for her age; her weight was 40.6 kilograms (89 lb), in the 50th percentile. The pediatrician noted some weight loss since Emily's previous visit and asked the family if any other symptoms were present. Emily's mother said that she had noted a 7-pound weight loss over 5 months, which she attributed to participation in competitive sports. Emily had also demonstrated an increase in thirst, but this was attributed to hot weather. No polyuria was noted. Laboratory analysis found glucose in the urine, but no ketones; a normal bicarbonate of 22 mEq/L; a normal pH; and a blood glucose of 456 mg/dL. Emily was diagnosed with Type 1 diabetes.

CASE STUDY.   Bobby K. was 11 years old when he noted nocturia, followed about 2 weeks later by polydipsia. For a day or two he complained of headache and dizziness. Bobby had an 18-year-old brother who had been diagnosed with Type 1 diabetes 5 years previously. His parents, familiar with the diagnosis and management of Type 1 diabetes, checked his urine, which showed 2 percent glucose and negative ketones. They also checked a fasting blood glucose, using one of his brother's meters. It was 194 mg/dL. But a check the next day by Bobby's pediatrician showed a postprandial blood glucose of 408 mg/dL. This was no surprise to Bobby or his parents. Diagnosis by parents is not unusual, especially when there is another child in the family or a close relative with Type 1 diabetes. (In general, however, meters should not be used by anyone but the person for whom they were prescribed, because of the risk of spreading blood-borne infections such as hepatitis and human immunodeficiency virus. Also, if two people share a meter, there is the potential of confusing one person's readings with the other's.)

As the above cases illustrate, diagnosis often depends upon the awareness and astuteness of the primary care clinician and the family.

The classic symptoms of Type 1 diabetes include

> ➤ polyuria;
> ➤ polydipsia;
> ➤ polyphagia, although not as predictable as the first two symptoms; and
> ➤ weight loss.

Other symptoms may indicate diabetes but may also be attributed to other pediatric causes. The young child who was previously dry at night and begins to wet the bed may have diabetes. Weight loss or failure to gain weight normally may be attributed to a panoply of conditions, but diabetes should always be considered.

Polyuria is often a prominent feature of Type 1 diabetes because, as blood glucose increases above the renal threshold and glucose spills into the urine, the glucose pulls water with it (an osmotic effect), leading to increased urine volume. Assessment of hydration is an important consideration in diagnosing diabetes, but signs of hydration can easily be misinterpreted. For example, if a young child has an illness with vomiting, the pediatrician, in a phone consultation, will ask the parent if the child is drinking and urinating. If the answer is yes, this may provide false assurance that there is no dehydration. However, if the child has diabetes, she may be drinking and putting out urine and still be very dehydrated. In the case of children with diabetes, using urine output as a measure of hydration status can be misleading, and urine output should be taken into account along with other factors such as weight loss, and moist versus dry mucosa. Diabetes must be considered in any child who is clinically dehydrated while continuing to urinate regularly.

The majority of children with new-onset Type 1 diabetes have symptoms of less than 1 month's duration. Others will experience mild to moderate symptoms over a period of several months. Questions about bed wetting, the number of diapers used, nocturia, and how often the child leaves the classroom to use the bathroom during the day may help to uncover polyuria.

The diagnosis is more likely to be missed in young children and infants in the early stages of the disease because of the difficulty of recognizing the early symptoms of polyuria and polydypsia. Consequently, very young children are more likely to present in ketoacidosis.

Primary care clinicians should have a very low threshold of suspicion to justify checking the urine for glucose and ketones. If the diagnosis of diabetes is not made and treatment is not begun, the child's condition is likely to worsen, often rapidly. Routine dipstick testing for urine glucose and ketones in patients with nonspecific symptoms such as lethargy, weight loss, nausea, and vomiting, as well as those with more classic diabetes symptoms, would facilitate the early diagnosis of this disease before severe metabolic decompensation has occurred. Also, with dipstick testing, results should be immediately available.

While the diagnostic criteria are usually clear-cut, two additional cases illustrate the difficulty of making a diagnosis when the symptoms are not immediately definitive.

> CASE STUDY.   Alan B. presented incidentally. At age 9, he was found to have positive urine glucose on a routine urinalysis, with a corresponding blood glucose of 222 mg/dL. He had no symptoms. Six hours later, his blood glucose was 308, his pH was 7.43, and his bicarbonate was 26 mEq/L, within the normal range.
>
> Alan was admitted to the hospital, and additional laboratory work showed a glycohemoglobin of 7.3 percent (normal range: 4.5 to 6.1%) with negative anti-insulin antibodies and negative islet cell antibodies. During his 2-day hospital admission, all additional blood glucose levels were normal, after the initial two high counts. Alan was educated about diabetes and was shown how to inject insulin and self-monitor but was not started on insulin in the hospital. He was sent home with instructions for twice-daily monitoring. His only diet restriction was to avoid simple sugar.
>
> In the next 6 months, Alan's glycohemoglobin returned to normal and his blood glucose levels were mostly in the 70 to 140 mg/dL range. He remained symptom-free. Then a glucose tolerance test showed normal fasting blood glucose levels but elevated levels after oral glucose, with a peak of 223 at 1 hour. Glycohemoglobin levels increased to slightly above normal. Outpatient monitoring showed predinner blood glucose levels that increased gradually over a period of months.
>
> In a 3-month period, between 6 to 9 months after initial presentation, Alan's weight decreased by 1.2 kilograms and his glycohemoglobin increased to 10 percent. He was then started on insulin.

The many months of waiting to see how things would progress for Alan made this a difficult situation for his family. It might have been easier for Alan's family if his diagnosis had been clear-cut from the beginning. Because the laboratory tests were not definitive, however, the family was slow to accept the diagnosis and the recommendation for insulin treatment, maintaining that if they controlled his diet and exercise he wouldn't have a blood glucose problem.

> **CASE STUDY.**   Leroy D. was also 9 years old when his diabetes first mani-fested itself in a manner similar to Alan's. A routine urinalysis showed glu-cose, but Leroy had no overt symptoms. A random blood glucose measure-ment was 125 mg/dL. Upon questioning, Leroy's mother remembered incidents of polyuria and polydipsia and one occasion of nocturia. He had also lost about 10 pounds over 1 month and had occasional headaches. His family doctor did an oral GTT, which showed a normal fasting glucose of 94 and postglucose levels that were all normal. Leroy's glycohemoglobin was also within the normal range.
>
> Leroy was put on a diet that avoided simple sugars. Six months later, he had a low blood glucose level of 57 mg/dL and was symptomatic, feeling lightheaded and dizzy. He was referred to an endocrinologist. An oral GTT showed a normal fasting glucose, but the 2-hour glucose was 203 (ele-vated). His glycohemoglobin was still normal.
>
> Leroy's physician thought that treating him with insulin might slow the autoimmune destructive process and help preserve the boy's beta cell func-tion. (For a further discussion of this theory, see the section on the Diabetes Prevention Trial in chapter 1.) Two months later, he was begun on Ultra-lente insulin twice a day. Because of continuing low morning blood glu-cose levels (below 70 mg/dL), the family stopped the evening Ultralente af-ter 2 months and just continued with the morning dose.
>
> They came to our clinic for a second opinion when Leroy was 11 years old. Leroy's mother was very confused about whether her son had diabetes or not. He was 144 centimeters (56.7 in.) tall and weighed 43 kilograms (95 lb), in the 50th and 85th percentiles, respectively. Within 9 months, Leroy was on full insulin doses, as his home monitoring showed a gradual pattern of elevated blood glucose levels and our testing found his glycohemoglobin levels rising in concert with his home blood glucose readings.

In both of the above cases, the team explained to the families of the boys that they were progressively losing beta cell function (i.e., were on the downslope of the curve shown in fig. 1.1). Although there may be some un-usual people who start down that slope but stop before the development of any overt disease, exhibiting only mild glucose intolerance, these are probably uncommon. In most cases, once clinical symptoms are seen, the child will progress to overt Type 1 diabetes.

There are other forms of hyperglycemia that are not due to beta cell destruction, and these are usually more transient than Type 1 diabetes. They include stress hyperglycemia, or hyperglycemia caused by fever or an infectious disease. These occur when illnesses cause the body to release stress hormones, which counter the action of insulin. Also, prednisone and related drugs in high doses can cause hyperglycemia, as do other drugs, including diazoxide, dilantin, thiazides, beta-adrenergics, and alpha-interferon. As noted above, children with cystic fibrosis may also develop diabetes. The diabetes of children with cystic fibrosis is usually easier to manage than classic Type 1 diabetes because insulin production does not cease altogether. Theories of management for children with cystic fibrosis are changing as other medical advances have lengthened these patients' life spans and necessitated more aggressive diabetes management to try to prevent long-term diabetes complications.

INITIAL MANAGEMENT

For patients who are obviously sick, the first medical goal of management is to stabilize them and treat ketoacidosis. (Ketoacidosis is discussed in detail in chapter 10.) After any acute problems have been treated, there are two major goals in the first few days after the initial diagnosis of Type 1 diabetes: (1) to teach the child and the family what they need to know about diabetes so that they can safely manage it; and (2) to establish a reasonable dosage of insulin, on the basis of the child's age, size, level of physical activity, and caloric intake or meal plan.

Whether or not to hospitalize the patient is a controversial question, and philosophies differ among practitioners. Some differences are geographic and depend upon the quality and availability of intensive outpatient management and education programs and home health care services. The attitudes and abilities of the parents are also important factors. While the criteria for hospitalization can be flexible, there are some clear-cut guidelines. If the child has DKA or another life-threatening condition, hospitalization is imperative.

Most families need the medical and psychological support that comes with hospitalization. It is the experience of our team, after dealing with children with diabetes and their families for many years, that the chronicity of this disease, the complexity of its care, and its impact on so many aspects of personal and family life make it risky to diagnose children and not admit them. Hospitalization may not be necessary if the family already has a child with Type 1 diabetes and is knowledgeable about management, or if a daytime hospital-like intensive management and education program is available. Usually, hospitalizing the patient for at least a couple of days will allow professionals to address the wide array of needs that the family of a newly diagnosed child with Type 1 diabetes will find confronting them, by providing

> ➤ detailed demonstrations of the required regimens for child and family;
> ➤ education about all aspects of Type 1 diabetes, especially survival skills;
> ➤ a chance to have their questions answered in depth; and
> ➤ an opportunity for clinicians to observe how well the family is handling this new complication in their lives.

There are two major educational pathways that must be addressed concurrently. The first is technical. Before a child leaves the hospital, he and his family must have all the necessary supplies in place (detailed in chapter 3) and must know

> ➤ how to check blood glucose;
> ➤ how to check urine ketones;
> ➤ how to draw up different insulins into the syringe and inject them;
> ➤ what to eat and when to eat it;
> ➤ what are the symptoms of high and low blood glucose;
> ➤ what to do when these symptoms occur, and how to treat highs and lows;
> ➤ when to call for help, and whom to call; and
> ➤ how to use glucagon.

The second pathway is cognitive, and it can be even more difficult. It requires grasping the principles of determining how much and what types of insulin are needed and understanding how insulin and food and exercise work together. This is the goal of "thinking like a pancreas"—something few families will have fully mastered by the time they leave the hospital, but they should be moving toward it.

Generally, the child who is not in DKA will be started on twice-a-day insulin, a combination of NPH (Neutral Protamine Hagedorn) insulin and a short-acting insulin (either Regular or lispro [Humalog]) before breakfast and again before dinner. Regular insulin begins to act about 30 to 60 minutes after injection, peaks 2 to 4 hours later, and lasts a total of 4 to 8 hours. Lispro begins to act about 15 minutes after injection, peaks at about 30 to 60 minutes, and lasts about 3 to 4 hours. These durations are quite variable from patient to patient, and even vary at different times in the same patient. NPH is absorbed into the body more slowly. It lasts an average of 13 hours, with peak activity 6 to 8 hours after injection. Ultralente is a third form of insulin, lasting about 18 hours and having more consistent action, without much of a peak.

A general formula for determining initial insulin doses is to have the number of units equal three-quarters of the child's weight in kilograms. Of this total, two-thirds is given in the morning and one-third before dinner, with the split between NPH and Regular 2:1 or 1:1. For example, if a child weighs 40 kilograms, the maximum total insulin dose will be 30 units. Twenty units will be given in the morning and 10 in the evening, and each dose will be two-thirds NPH and one-third Regular, or one-half NPH and one-half Regular. Insulin types, action, and dosage are covered in detail in chapter 6.

If the newly diagnosed child is hospitalized, the length of hospitalization will vary according to the family's competence, the benefits provided by the family's health insurer or health maintenance organization, and the resources (e.g., hospital-based outpatient clinics and home health care services) that are available in the area. Some health plans may provide more comprehensive benefits for hospitalized patients. The necessary tasks can be accomplished with nearly all families in less than a week.

Once the child is off intravenous treatment and ready to start subcutaneous insulin, she can usually be discharged from the hospital in 2 or 3 days. Our hospital team (and many others) has developed a critical pathway to medical and educational goals that covers 2 nights and 3 days of hospitalization subsequent to conversion to subcutaneous insulin. A version of this is reproduced in Appendix H. Unless there are barriers to the completion of the critical pathway goals, the child can then be discharged.

Following discharge, an intermediate period of home education to reinforce what was taught in the hospital is a helpful and necessary transition for most families. Home care can be an extremely useful component of treatment until the child and family are ready to move completely into outpatient treatment.

The role of the primary care clinician during the period of hospitalization is variable, depending upon factors such as the type of hospital, the practitioner's personal relationship with the family, and the family's distance from the hospital. In a rural hospital, the primary care physician is likely to be the attending physician. In a large medical center, the specialty team will be attending, and the primary care clinician is likely to have a lesser role. However, the primary care clinician should remain in contact with the team and with the family throughout the hospitalization.

THE "HONEYMOON" PERIOD

After the initial presentation, most children and adolescents newly diagnosed with Type 1 diabetes undergo a remission phase, referred to as the "honeymoon" period. During this time, the remaining functional beta cells regain some of their ability to produce insulin. This may be a result of the correction of the hyperglycemia. Measurement of C-peptide levels (a reflection of endogenous insulin) has documented the improved insulin secretion that occurs during this phase.

Because of the increase of endogenous insulin secretion, requirements for exogenous insulin decrease, usually to less than 0.5 unit per kilogram of body weight per day. Hypoglycemia, therefore, is a potential problem, and close contact between the family and the clinician is very important during this period.

The honeymoon period usually begins within 1 to 3 months after diagnosis and lasts for several months, and occasionally as long as 1 or 2 years. For the patient, it is a period of relative well-being and metabolic normalcy, confirmed by near-normal glycohemoglobin levels. It is important that newly diagnosed patients and their families be educated about this honeymoon phenomenon. Unless they expect the occurrence of this phase and appreciate that it will not last forever, it may lead to denial of the disease and failure to monitor adequately.

As the honeymoon phase draws to a close, the remaining beta cells lose their capacity to secrete insulin, and the patient's requirements for exogenous insulin rise. Usually this occurs gradually, but occasionally, as with an acute infection, it may occur abruptly. Careful monitoring and frequent dose adjustments are extremely important during the end of the honeymoon period, and close contact between the patient and the clinician is necessary.

The honeymoon is a time for families to get accustomed to the Type 1 diabetes regimen and its demands on lifestyle. As the honeymoon ends and blood glucose rises, there may be a tendency for the parents (or the child or teenager himself) to blame the patient for eating sweets or not following the prescribed regimen correctly. It is important for families to understand that the elevated blood glucose levels as the honeymoon period ends are *not* anyone's fault and that no one should be blamed for them. The case of James T. shows the way in which insulin needs decrease during the honeymoon and then start to increase.

CASE STUDY.   James T. first developed polyuria, polydipsia, blurred vision, and fatigue at age 12 years. He was 155 centimeters (5 ft, 1 in.) in height and 45 kilograms (99 lb) in weight; his height and weight were both in the 75th percentile for his age. He was hospitalized with a blood glucose level of 533 mg/dL, normal pH, normal bicarbonate, and negative urine ketones. He was started on an insulin dose of 13 units of NPH and 8 units of Regular in the morning, and 4 units of NPH and 4 units of Regular in the evening. Three weeks after diagnosis, on the basis of his blood glucose levels, his insulin dose was decreased to 7 units of NPH (and no Regular) in the morning, and 2 units of NPH (and no Regular) in the evening. When he was on the previous doses, his blood glucose levels had been running normal to low.

Two months after diagnosis, James was still on the low insulin dose. Within 3 months, however, on the basis of continuing blood glucose monitoring, his insulin dose was gradually increased, and by 9 months after diagnosis, his morning dose was up to 8 units of NPH and 1 unit of Regular, and his evening dose was up to 8 units of NPH and 1 to 5 units of Regular. The dose continued to gradually increase. One year later (21 months after diagnosis), James had a glycohemoglobin in the target range. His insulin dose was up to 16 units of NPH and 2 to 4 units of Regular in the morning, and the same in the evening.

PSYCHOLOGICAL ISSUES

While mastery of the concepts underlying Type 1 diabetes care and the technical knowledge required for diabetes management can seem consuming for patients, families, and practitioners, it is also important not to ignore the psychological issues that accompany the diagnosis of this disease. When meeting with the family of a newly diagnosed child—even if it is not the first child in the family with diabetes—the primary care clinician should always address the emotional impact of this chronic disease on a child or teenager who had previously seemed healthy.

After telling families and patients what to expect medically, we counsel them that this is an extremely stressful time. Many people feel overwhelmed and frightened. People's needs are different. Some require a great deal of support from their clinicians and some require less, and the amount of support they need may not be directly related to their level of education, the adequacy of their other support systems, or any other predictable factors. We ask families to try to let us know if they feel that there is some information or service they need but are not receiving. Part of the reason for hospitalization of the newly diagnosed child is to enable these psychological issues to be addressed from the start, and to enable families to become easily and quickly acquainted with the range of services and personnel, both inpatient and outpatient, that are available for them when certain needs occur.

Shortly after diagnosis, it is important to tell families in detail what they can expect to happen over the next few days, and then project to the next few weeks and beyond. They must understand that despite the intensive training they will receive, their control of this disease will not be perfect when they leave the hospital. Diabetes management is complex and imperfect. It is quite normal for families to feel angry and sad. If these feelings are interfering with their ability to accomplish the goals of disease management, the clinician can assist in connecting them with appropriate psychological counseling services to help them understand and overcome these problems.

It is also important for the primary care clinician to recognize the depths of the sadness and anger and loss of control that many families will feel after hearing a diagnosis of diabetes and an explanation of its implications for family life. Another emotion families will be grappling with is fear—fear, first of all, about the immediate health of the child, and then fear about long-term health problems, and finally fear about whether they will be able to master the techniques, information, and skills they need to learn to treat diabetes.

You can assure families that by the time their new-onset diabetes education program is complete, they will know what they need to know for home management. In addition, home health care may be available for support, although this availability will depend on health insurance provisions and what the family can afford. It is helpful to discuss the specifics of reimbursement issues; for example, if their insurer or health maintenance organization authorizes only a certain pharmacy for prescriptions, they may not be able to get their diabetes supplies at the hospital pharmacy.

In addition to addressing the immediate psychological impact of the diabetes diagnosis on the family, it is also important to give the family an idea of what this will mean to them on a more long-term basis, and to give them an idea of how their lives will change. The changes will be considerable, in a number of different contexts. Families will find themselves involved in health care services as never before, seeing care providers on a regular and frequent basis and remaining in close contact between visits, especially at the beginning. The diagnosis of diabetes may have effects on both health insurance and life insurance coverage. Families will be confronted with a regimen of tasks that must be performed every day, requiring a daily time commitment, which may truly present a challenge in the busy lives of parents, especially in single-parent or dual-career families.

But the biggest change they will have to face is the need for planning for every occasion, the difficulty of spontaneity. No longer can they pile the family into the car and say, "We're off on a day trip." Now they must pack medical and food supplies, plan for contingencies (e.g., getting stuck in traffic), and think through their plans from beginning to end, making sure that the needs of the child with diabetes will not be overlooked. The same is true of any other means of travel. We recommend that patients who are going on an airplane trip pack two sets of supplies in case of loss or theft: one set that is checked with their luggage and a second that they carry with them or that is carried by another person who is traveling with them. Each set should include insulin, syringes, monitoring equipment, and glucagon. The child with diabetes should always carry a sugar source on his or her person.

The risks of not planning properly are illustrated by the following case studies:

> CASE STUDY.   Shawn L. is only 14½ years old, but he is already an experienced and accomplished golfer. Diagnosed with diabetes when he was 9 months old, he has known the need for control and management his whole life, but a recent experience reinforced for him the need to always plan for contingencies.
>
> At the time of this event, Shawn was in midpuberty, 167 centimeters (5 ft, 6½ in.) tall and weighing 56 kilograms (121 lb), in the 75th and 60th percentiles, respectively, for his age. His insulin dosage was 34 units of NPH

and 4 to 10 units of Regular in the morning, and 26 units of NPH and 1 to 6 units of Regular in the evening. He had a history of variable control—sometimes good, sometimes suboptimal.

Shawn left for the golf course in the morning with his father after taking his insulin and eating only a small breakfast. His plan was to eat at the snack bar on the golf course, but it was closed. With only a few crackers to counterbalance the insulin, he had a serious hypoglycemic reaction. He felt himself getting low and becoming disoriented and then belligerent. His father called 911, and when the emergency medical technicians arrived on the scene they administered intravenous glucose. Shawn was taken to a local emergency department, where he was treated and released. When he later described the event to us, he acknowledged that he had ignored what he had learned in his years of managing his condition. "It didn't turn out to be a very good day for golf," he said.

CASE STUDY.   Julie F. was 16 years old when she went camping with her family on a remote island that could only be reached by boat. Managing diabetes was not new to her; she had been diagnosed at age 4. However, poor planning left her without glucagon to treat a hypoglycemic seizure.

Camping with her parents and two sisters, Julie—who was postpubertal, with height and weight both in the 50th percentile—engaged in a great deal of physical exercise, including canoeing on the river. She ate dinner and a snack and was fine when she went to sleep, although she did not monitor her blood glucose level. In the morning, before breakfast, she had a seizure. Her family had not included glucagon with their camping supplies, although they did have a tube of cake icing on hand. However, it took them nearly an hour to carefully squeeze enough icing into Julie's mouth (being careful to avoid aspiration) for her condition to normalize. In this case, no emergency rescue was needed, but as soon as Julie was stable the family left the island, cutting short their vacation.

These incidents illustrate why it is vitally important to carry supplies and to plan, *plan* ahead.

CASE STUDY.   Alex D. is 8 years old and was diagnosed with diabetes when he was 5. His glycemic control is good, and he is able to sense approaching lows and quickly treat them. "I just grab anything I can get my hands on and eat it," Alex reported during a clinic visit. Rather offhandedly, during the visit, Alex's mother mentioned that the family was planning a trip to Disney World in about 3 weeks.

Alex can have as good a time at Disney World as any other child, but there are important points to remember and steps to take to prevent problems on his vacation. Remember, we warned Alex and his mother, that the lines for food can be very long. He should take a backpack with lots of snacks and sugar. "On the day that we do the water park, he'll be jumping around a lot," his mother noted. We decided together that on his active days at the park, Alex should decrease his NPH doses by 10 to 20 percent and supplement with Regular if he needed it to cover calories and carbohydrates.

PRACTICAL POINTS FOR CLINICIANS

1. Have a low threshold for checking urine or blood glucose and/or urine ketones. Think of Type 1 diabetes not only when you see classic Type 1 diabetes symptoms but also in instances of weight loss, lethargy, and vomiting or nausea.

2. You can manage new-onset Type 1 diabetes in either an inpatient or outpatient setting, depending on the severity of metabolic decompensation, the available health care resources, and the abilities of the patient and family.

3. Newly diagnosed patients and their families need both technical and cognitive education and skills.

4. Families need to be educated about the psychological implications of the diabetes diagnosis, and its impact on family life.

5. Patients and families must learn to plan ahead.

3

Survival Skills for Patients and Parents

To begin to master all the various components that are involved in diabetes management, it is necessary to consider all the factors that affect blood glucose levels: the type, quantity, and timing of insulin, of food, of exercise and other physical activity, and of stress. Once diabetes is diagnosed and the child is medically stable, the family can start on the road to successfully mastering the concepts of initial management and the specific details of the "survival skills" that are necessary for living with diabetes. As they learn the rationale and how-to of the survival skills, families will begin to understand that this is a disease that must be managed primarily in the home, not in the clinician's office.

The survival skills fall into five categories:

➤ giving (and preparing for) insulin injections;
➤ monitoring blood glucose and urine ketones, and recordkeeping;
➤ food management, including meal plans;
➤ exercise management; and
➤ management of acute problems, especially hypoglycemia.

These should be taught in the hospital before the patient is discharged from an inpatient program, or in the first days of an outpatient program. But families must understand that proficiency will come only with continued practice and understanding of the principles and responsibilities involved in managing diabetes. Psychological issues—discussed in detail in chapter 11—are also important to consider from the earliest stages of diabetes care. A number of books and other publications are available to help families with all of these topics; several are listed in Appendix I, "Resources." We recommend initial daily telephone contact between clinicians and newly diagnosed patients and their families, with gradual weaning as the patients and families learn to master the regimen. This weaning period can range from a couple of weeks to a few months.

INSULIN INJECTIONS

At least one parent and the child, if old enough, will need to learn how to inject insulin. How old is old enough? This is a logical question, but there is no definitive answer because children have such a variable range of development and cognitive ability. In the case of prekindergarten children, most of the education is directed at the parents, with simple explanations provided for the children. By the age of about 10 years, almost all children are able to take charge of the actual injections themselves, and the specifics of this education will be directed at them. Often, both parents, as well as grandparents and older siblings, will also want to learn how to inject insulin, and it is helpful if more than one family member is schooled in this continuing task.

Learning how to inject insulin includes learning what insulins are available, how they work, and their timing of action. Caregivers must understand which insulin has which duration of action and covers which time of the day. This is explained in detail in chapter 6.

The first step in injecting insulin is to gather the necessary supplies. Insulin, a syringe, a cotton swab, and alcohol are needed. It is important to check that the insulin is not outdated. Once a vial has been opened, it should be kept no longer than 3 months. It is best if insulin is at room temperature when injected. If it has been refrigerated, it may be brought to room temperature. Refrigeration of the vial that is in use is not usually necessary. Studies have found that insulin stored at room temperature loses only 1.5 percent of its potency per month, which would not have a significant impact on its efficacy. It should be kept in a cool place, and away from direct sunlight. Extra vials should be refrigerated.

If insulin is kept at temperatures above 90 degrees Fahrenheit or below freezing, it will lose potency. If, in long-acting insulin, there are clumps sticking to the side of the bottle, or if, in Regular insulin, the solution is cloudy, the medication is probably spoiled and should be discarded.

Once supplies have been gathered, the next step is to accurately measure insulin into the syringe. When the dose is a combination of short-acting (Regular or lispro) and long-acting insulins, the short-acting insulin is traditionally drawn up into the syringe first, in order to not contaminate the Regular or lispro with longer-acting insulin and thus change the timing of the drug action of the shorter-acting insulin. The long-acting insulin should then be drawn up, after the vial is rolled or gently shaken so that the insulin is mixed.

It is important that parents and children know the total dose of insulin for each injection and that they double-check their addition, so that the correct total amount is drawn up. When the child is giving the injections, drawing up the correct amount must be carefully supervised. Children in a hurry sometimes draw up more air than insulin. Another important point to make clear to concerned parents and patients is that even though air bubbles will lower the actual insulin dose delivered, they cause no harm to the patient.

Insulin injections are given subcutaneously. It is helpful for patients and their parents to have a diagram of possible injection sites. These include the upper arms, thighs, abdomen, and buttocks. Insulin is absorbed most quickly from the abdomen, followed by the arms, then the thighs, and then the buttocks. In the past, to prevent the development of atrophy or hypertrophy of subcutaneous fat, the rotation of injection sites was recommended. The newer, highly purified insulins make atrophy or hypertrophy much less of a problem. Because of the variability of absorption characteristics for different sites, we now often recommend, for consistency of absorption, that patients remain with one site for a period of time lasting up to several weeks, and then move to another. Sometimes we suggest that patients use one site for morning injections and another for evening injections, so that, for example, the child is injecting in his arm in the morning and in his thigh at night. For each site, the child rotates the shot over that whole area.

Once the site has been selected, the person administering the injection should clean the site carefully with alcohol on a cotton swab or with soap and water, pinch the skin, and insert the needle. Some suggest holding the needle at a 90-degree angle, others at a 45-degree angle; we have found that either angle works well, and the patient should choose what feels comfortable for her. For a small child with minimal body fat, a 45-degree angle may be the best. The child or parent should push the needle all the way in. Making sure that the needle is still all the way in, the child or parent should push the plunger slowly and smoothly, as far as it will go. If leakage is a problem, he or she should let go of the pinch and wait 5 to 10 seconds before withdrawing the needle. Leakage can cause the loss of a significant amount of insulin and is a common reason for variability in blood glucose levels.

The injection hurts, but it doesn't hurt much. However, every clinician who works with children knows that fear of needles can be extremely anxiety-producing for many patients. There is considerable variability from child to child. For some, getting an injection is a terrifying experience. Others find the whole process very interesting and quickly learn to take charge of the injections themselves, welcoming the "grown-up" feeling. Some will say that sometimes the shots hurt and sometimes they don't hurt at all. That may be a function of technique, luck, or success in getting the child's mind on another subject. Many children grow out of the feeling of fearing injections. Eddie J. is a good example.

CASE STUDY.   Eddie J. is 4 years old and was diagnosed with diabetes when he was 18 months old. Since the diagnosis, giving him his injections has been a continuing ordeal for his grandparents, who are his caretakers. For 3 years, injection time meant screaming and thrashing and tears, even though blood glucose monitoring was not a problem. Suddenly, though, a few months after he turned 4, Eddie began to accept the twice-daily insulin injections as a necessary part of his life. Now, at injection time, he'll dutifully lay himself across his grandfather's lap and count to 10. The injection comes at about "8," and a minute later Eddie will spring back up to whatever he had been doing.

Children who are frightened by needles should be handled gently, without bullying. No child should be forced to inject herself until she is psychologically ready. In our experience, this is rarely a problem in older children, once they have discussed the issues, gone over the techniques and routine, and been permitted to vent their feelings.

Air-pressure injectors are an alternative to needles, although we have encountered some problems when they are used. Some children complain that they hurt. Trying to adjust to appropriate pressure settings may cause leakage of insulin. However, the latest generation of these devices is considerably improved over earlier models, and they may be of benefit to very young children or children with a genuine phobia about needles.

MONITORING AND RECORDKEEPING

Blood Glucose Monitoring

Blood glucose monitoring is the cornerstone of diabetes management. The primary educational goals for clinicians dealing with the newly diagnosed child or adolescent with diabetes include teaching the child and the family how to monitor and record results, seeing what the blood glucose levels are, and beginning to help the family understand how to move the blood glucose into the target range.

All of the other variables of diabetes control—insulin dosage, food intake, and amount of physical activity—must be measured and balanced according to what the blood glucose monitoring indicates. For the past two decades, the availability of the technology necessary to provide accurate and nearly instant readings of blood glucose levels has changed the lives of people with diabetes, giving them the means to manage their disease in a way never before possible. Children and adolescents with diabetes can use the information obtained from monitoring to understand how different foods and physical activities affect them, make the appropriate insulin adjustments, and take control of their disease.

It is important that families understand that the goal of monitoring for every patient and family (and health care provider) is to get to know the patient's disease. This is a very individualized thing. What is the blood glucose response to different insulins at various times of the day? What are the durations of different insulins? When are they likely to peak, and when are they likely to wear off? How does exercise affect blood glucose? What do different foods do to blood glucose? The only way to get answers to these questions is to monitor blood glucose levels.

The more frequently monitoring is done, the more information you will have, and the better decisions you will be able to make about the adjustments that are necessary to get blood glucose—and therefore glycohemoglobins—into the target range. Monitoring several times a day is imperative in order to truly know what must be done to adjust the regimen. This information about how and when to make adjustments will allow flexibility in the life of the child or teen with diabetes. In general, monitoring should be done before an injection and before a meal, so that the information about the glucose level can influence the dose decision and meal content.

There are two means of looking at the amount of glucose in the blood. Self-monitoring of blood glucose is the narrowly focused snapshot, providing several daily (even hourly, if needed) status reports on the amount of glucose in the blood. Glycohemoglobin is a more long-term measurement showing a bigger picture. It measures the glucose attached to hemoglobin, reflecting a longer term of control. The attachment of glucose to the hemoglobin molecule is an irreversible action; the glucose remains attached for the life of the cell. Red blood cells live for about 4 months, and glycohemoglobin measurements therefore reflect blood glucose levels over a 2- to 3-month period. Glycohemoglobin is measured in most laboratories. The details of monitoring glycohemoglobin are explained in chapter 4.

It is crucial that children with diabetes and their families have the right attitude about these important gauges. Blood glucose and glycohemoglobin levels are *not* report cards. They are measurements that provide important and necessary information that will help the patient, the family, and the health care provider achieve the best control possible over this disease. Research shows that frequent monitoring correlates with improved glucose control, which in turn means fewer long-term complications for children and adolescents with diabetes.

However, families must also recognize that management of this difficult disease cannot be flawless or absolute. They should not let perfect be the enemy of good. A reasonable and attainable goal is to aim for 75 to 80 percent of blood glucose counts in the target range. This will usually produce an acceptable glycohemoglobin level.

It is also important for families and health care providers to recognize that at various times in any individual's life, even this short-of-perfection goal may be too burdensome to be carried. People sometimes need to step back from this disease for short periods of time. There may be times when, because of psychosocial issues, the medical goals temporarily become secondary to the goals of trying to achieve a psychologically healthy and balanced lifestyle. Compromises may be needed, weighing the total life of the child or adolescent against the constant demands of diabetes control. If a person's entire energy goes into diabetes control, he could have near-perfect control but an incomplete and unhappy life. It is necessary to find a balance, and to recognize that this balance is a moving target that will shift at various ages. Dealing with this is up to the individual and family who are coping with diabetes. Ultimately, it is not the role of doctors, nurses, or dietitians to demand or compel certain behaviors. What the clinician can do is know the range of issues, the spectrum of choices, the risks and benefits of each choice, and the individual needs of each patient.

> CASE STUDY.   Chuck R. is 16 years old and just got his driver's license. He wants to go out for Coke and pizza with his friends at 10 P.M. Chuck and his parents know that two slices of pizza, if not covered with insulin, will raise Chuck's overnight blood glucose to more than 400 mg/dL. Chuck has a number of choices: (1) not to go out with his friends; (2) to go out with his friends and have diet Coke and a low-fat salad; (3) to go out with his friends and eat what he wants, injecting Regular insulin to cover his calories and carbohydrates just before eating; or (4) not to bother with the insulin, eat what he wants, and just let the blood glucose rise over 400.

While the fourth alternative means the least control at this point in time and is the least satisfactory choice for metabolic control, sometimes this may seem the best option to a teenager who wants to normalize his life and not feel different from his peers. Symptoms of hyperglycemia may help Chuck decide against this alternative, and he needs to know that repeated occurrences of hyperglycemia would definitely pose long-term risks and that this option should only rarely be considered. But one incident of high blood glucose at this level does not represent an acute risk and may be acceptable for Chuck to choose in the context of everything else that is going on in his life at this time.

Self-monitoring involves poking, or lancing, the finger for a drop of blood. Several different lancets are commercially available, and some have variable depth settings, allowing blood to be drawn from the minimum depth possible. Superfine lancets may be less painful than thicker lancets. A drop of blood is put on a pad, or on a strip in the glucose meter. A number of different meters to measure blood glucose are available, and each has slightly different instructions for use. It should be emphasized again that a monitor should only be used by the person it is prescribed for, so that there is no risk of spreading blood-borne diseases or confusing readings.

We recommend that our patients self-monitor for blood glucose about four times each day. Shortly after diagnosis, while the insulin dosage is still being determined, more than four daily measurements will be necessary, including some measurements taken during the overnight hours. More frequent monitoring may also be necessary for younger children who have a difficult time communicating information about symptoms they may be experiencing, and is needed whenever the child (of any age) is sick. Until the regimen is mastered, patients and families should have frequent contact with the clinician, initially calling or faxing in the results of blood glucose monitoring every day.

The target blood glucose range is somewhat discretionary, depending on the age of the child, the time of day, and attitudes about management. The initial goal will be to achieve blood glucose levels below 200 mg/dL. This will be refined as control is mastered. Ideally, the target will be between 70 and 120 mg/dL, with an upper level of 120 before meals and 180 about 2 hours after meals. More reasonable goals are 70 to 180 for schoolchildren and 70 to 150 for teens. A range of 100 to 200 is acceptable for babies and toddlers, because of their inability to communicate symptoms and their risk of hypoglycemia. Bedtime levels should be higher, generally 100 to 140, although this level may need to be raised if the child has had more exercise and/or less food intake on a specific day, or if the child's blood glucose is known to decrease significantly overnight. The nadir overnight (between 2 A.M. and 4 A.M.) should be above 70 to 80, and perhaps above 100 for babies and toddlers.

However, if a child or adolescent is usually in the target range but sometimes has significantly low blood glucose (below 60 mg/dL) and/or hypoglycemic symptoms, this is not ideal, and the high-end goals should be loosened. Some children are able to maintain levels very close to normal without significant hypoglycemia, while others develop bothersome symptoms at these levels. It is not possible to predict who will be in this latter group, and this underscores the need for intensive individualized management of each diabetes patient by the family and clinician.

Although it can be difficult to predict who will have trouble with monitoring, some indicators should be heeded. Dysfunctional families, families in which the child and parents do not work together to achieve their goals, may have trouble with blood glucose management. Diabetes management may be more difficult with intense children or children who easily react to stress. Special attention must be given to children involved in athletics, who may need to markedly increase their caloric intake or significantly decrease their insulin doses on an exercise day to allow for the increased physical activity.

Overnight monitoring is periodically necessary, especially in the case of newly diagnosed patients and children or teens with management problems. All patients need to have blood glucose checked periodically in the middle of the night, usually between 2 A.M. and 4 A.M., when the evening dose of NPH is peaking. This is particularly important for children who have eaten less than usual, exercised more than usual, adjusted their insulin dose, or deviated in any way from their customary routine. Sometimes, when morning control continues to be inadequate, overnight blood glucose panels every 2 to 3 hours are necessary.

Ketone Monitoring

It is also very important for families to learn how and when to monitor urine for ketones. Urine ketones are products of the breakdown of fat, and they occur when fat stores are being used for energy. This happens primarily when there is not enough insulin to allow glucose to be used for energy. Ketones can also occur when food intake is too low to provide the energy needed. Nondiabetics will develop ketones when fasting for prolonged periods.

Ketones are an early sign of impending problems. It is important to check the urine for ketones to prevent ketoacidosis from occurring. Ketones are checked by a dipstick, and there are several types of dipsticks available. Ketones should be checked whenever the blood glucose is elevated, usually above 250 to 300 mg/dL. They should also be checked anytime a person with diabetes is sick, and especially when the person has an upset stomach, nausea, and/or vomiting. Ketones may be present when a person is ill, even without hyperglycemia. Ketone measurements are classified as negative, trace, small, moderate, or large. The timing of the reading of the strip must adhere to the manufacturer's instructions. Moderate to large ketones require additional insulin. In the period shortly following diagnosis, patients who find ketones should consult with the clinician to determine the necessary adjustment to their insulin dosage. Patients should continue to monitor trace to small ketones and consult with the clinician if they are persistent. This is often necessary when a child is ill, as in the case of Erica J. (See chapter 8 for more specifics on sick day management.)

> CASE STUDY.   Erica J. is 6 years old and weighs 25 kilograms (55 lb). She has had diabetes for 2 years. During an illness, with a temperature of 102.5 Fahrenheit and significant cough and nasal congestion, Erica's blood glucose level rose to 315 mg/dL, even though she had eaten very little. Her ketones were moderate. Her parents consulted with our office, and we in-

structed them to give Erica 2 to 3 units of Regular insulin every 3 to 4 hours until the ketones cleared and the blood glucose began to drop. We also advised them that it was important to cover the insulin with calories once the blood glucose level began to drop, and that Erica should drink extra fluid to prevent dehydration.

Recordkeeping

Recordkeeping is the critical adjunct to monitoring. It is very important to keep good records of blood glucose levels and insulin doses. The parents of children and adolescents with diabetes, and the patients themselves (when they are old enough), must understand the need to write down the results of each blood glucose check, as well as what insulin doses were given, sometimes what was eaten, and information about other variables. Recording this information allows quick detection of developing problems, accurate troubleshooting, and informed choices to make necessary adjustments. The more information you have, the better you will be able to adjust the variables if control is suboptimal.

New technology is making recordkeeping increasingly simple. Computer software programs are available which download the data recorded by the blood glucose meter and chart the information (see figs. 3.1 and 3.2). Even recording information by hand on a chart only takes seconds, and adequate recordkeeping can be accomplished in less than 5 minutes a day. However, we have found in our practice that some children hate keeping these records—it feels too much like homework. Often this can be handled by parceling out the responsibilities, with the child being responsible for remembering to actually do the finger-stick and reporting the results to the parent, who will then chart the numbers. Sample recordkeeping charts can be found in Appendixes B and C. But a multitude of family issues can be reflected in the problems that sometimes characterize recordkeeping, as the difficult case of Clifton H. illustrates.

CASE STUDY.   Clifton H. is 15 years old and has had an insulin pump for a year. He is in late puberty, is 165 centimeters (5 ft, 5 in.) tall, and weighs 51 kilograms (112 pounds), in the 25th percentile for his age for both height and weight. His father is a businessman and his mother an attorney, and they both frequently travel for their work. Clifton has been left alone to manage his diabetes since before he had the maturity to handle it, and his control through the years reflects this. His recordkeeping is indifferent. His

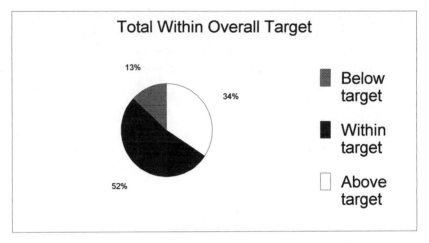

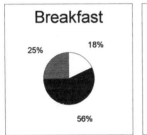 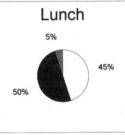 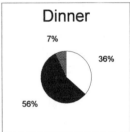

Fig. 3.1.   The percentage of blood glucose levels below, within, and above a target range at specific times of day, for the last 250 readings.
Figure generated by In-Touch Diabetes Management Software.

glycohemoglobin levels reflect a pattern of intermittent hyperglycemia, which has little effect on his current health but considerable negative implications for the future.

Clifton uses a meter with a memory that keeps track of his blood glucose levels, but he does not chart these numbers and does not keep track of his insulin doses or look at patterns. Therefore he does not learn when his dose decisions are appropriate or inappropriate. Overall, his control is suboptimal, with blood glucose levels above 200 mg/dL about 40 percent of the time and in the target range the rest of the time, and he could substantially improve his management if he looked at patterns and used this information to evaluate his dose decisions, with the supervision and input of one or both of his parents. As it is, it is very difficult to suggest regimen modifications for him without more information.

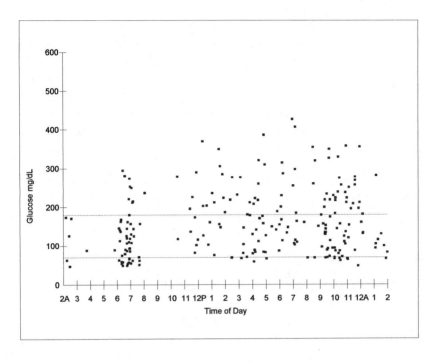

Overall Target Range

Fig. 3.2.   The range of blood glucose levels plotted for time of day, for the last 250 readings.
Figure generated by In-Touch Diabetes Management Software.

FOOD MANAGEMENT

In most families, eating is the most important continuing family ritual. Food restrictions or food preferences cause arguments in many families, even without the complexities of diabetes. Diabetes control centers around meal planning, and it is important that families have positive and constructive attitudes about integrating this phase of management into their everyday lives.

Appropriate vocabulary can help to set the tone. We recommend that this aspect of diabetes management *not* be referred to as "diet." *Diet* is a restrictive, confining term that implies limitations, self-denial, and hardship. A more positive vocabulary speaks of "meal planning," "food management," or "food strategy." Likewise, we don't use the word *cheating* to refer to eating something that is not in the meal plan. Eating something extra is not the same as copying from a friend during a test at school. Children and teens with diabetes should not be made to feel guilty about what they eat. Parents should not be expected to play the role of "food police."

Diabetes control encompasses a spectrum of philosophies about food. The spectrum has evolved and broadened as simple and accurate monitoring techniques have become available. Whichever philosophy is adopted, one guideline must be followed: all food intake must be planned to a certain extent, and accounted for. Most children and teenagers typically eat snacks on the run, not thinking about caloric or carbohydrate content or nutritional value, and certainly not thinking about how much insulin this snack requires. Such spontaneity is difficult to reconcile with the planning that is necessary for the child or teen with diabetes.

We recommend that families with children with diabetes follow a typical three-meal plan (breakfast, lunch, and dinner) with a midafternoon snack and a before-bedtime snack. In addition, a midmorning snack should be included in the meal plans for young children, to avoid lows due to morning insulin.

The more traditional philosophy about food is that the same amount of food, with fixed calorie and carbohydrate contents, should be ingested at the same time each day. The insulin dosage is also mostly fixed and is based on these calorie and carbohydrate counts. To allow for some diversity in meals and snacks, exchange lists provide a variety of alternative foods with similar caloric and carbohydrate content.

A newer philosophy is that although meals and snacks should be eaten at approximately the same time each day, it is not necessary to eat the same types and amounts of food at every meal. Instead, the person with diabetes must learn to adjust his insulin doses in relation to his blood glucose level and the calorie and carbohydrate content of the food that will be consumed. All children and adults who are on a multiple-injection regimen or on insulin pumps learn to adjust their doses as needed. However, it may be best to postpone this flexibility until after the patient and/or family have mastered the basics of managing this disease. There is so much to learn and understand at first that minimizing the number of variables can be helpful. With our newly diagnosed patients, we usually teach a fairly simple meal plan involving a list of exchanges, with the same amount of food at the same time every day. Once disease-management skills are mastered, it is easier to move on to a more flexible eating regimen.

In one case, food intake and insulin doses are basically the same every day, with some adjustments for exercise and blood glucose levels. In the other, insulin doses are determined according to food intake. To illustrate, a child on a fixed regimen will think, "This is what I need to eat, based on my blood glucose level and insulin dosage." A child on a more variable, multiple-shot regimen will calculate, "This is what I want to eat for lunch, this is how many carbohydrate grams it contains; therefore, this is the insulin dose I need." This latter approach more closely approximates the goal of "thinking like a pancreas." Eventually each patient (and family) can select the place on this spectrum of flexibility at which they feel most comfortable. It is our experience that families with lower educational levels often feel more comfortable with the less flexible, more concrete, and more repetitive regimens. Some families may choose a fixed amount of food for breakfast and lunch on school days, with a flexible amount for dinner and for all meals on weekends and holidays.

In most cases, daily food intake will consist of about 50 to 55 percent carbohydrates, 20 percent protein, and the remainder fat. Fat intake should be prudent, with most of the calories coming from polyunsaturated fats. This is discussed in detail in chapter 7.

Children with diabetes (and their families) may fear that they can never have a piece of cake or candy again. This is not the case. It is an outdated myth that foods with sugar are off-limits to a person with diabetes. While sweets should be eaten in moderation, children and adolescents with diabetes don't have to avoid simple sugars totally—they need to cover them with insulin, and learn to work them into their meal and snack plans to comply with their calorie and carbohydrate intake goals. We do not advise for or against the use of artificial sweeteners; we think that this decision is up to the individual family, although we are comfortable using them.

Most children or teenagers or families with diabetes will tell you that dietary restrictions are the worst part of living with diabetes. Moving toward a more flexible regimen generally helps people to feel more in control of their lives and, consequently, more in control of their disease. Unfortunately, there are some children who feel that no matter what options are available for them, diabetes is ruining their lives. They have a great deal of difficulty getting beyond the perception that they have a chronic disease that taints their whole life.

More often, though, they learn to adjust. Clinicians can help them to do so by directly confronting their negative feelings. We often ask children or teens, "How is life with diabetes treating you?" or sometimes, when indicated, "Do you feel that diabetes is ruining your life?" We are quick to refer patients for counseling when we sense intimations of these types of emotional problems. Sometimes, though, practical problem-solving can get to the root of difficult behavior, and relatively simple solutions can be remarkably effective, as the following anecdote illustrates.

> CASE STUDY.   Ellen L. is 10 years old and has had diabetes since she was 11 months of age. She is generally a sweet, even-tempered child. One day, visiting the doctor for a regular appointment, her mother revealed that the girl was becoming increasingly angry, throwing syringes and alcohol swabs. In a private meeting with Ellen, the physician talked to her about her feelings. "You've had diabetes for a long time, and one of the things that happens to people with diabetes is that they get very angry about always having it," the doctor said. Large tears ran down Ellen's cheeks, and the doctor knew that she was on the right track. She then asked the girl, "What is the hardest thing for you about having diabetes?"
>
> "Not eating Oreo cookies," Ellen answered promptly.
>
> "Okay," the physician responded, "let's work out a plan. How many Oreo cookies do you think you need?"
>
> Two Oreo cookies twice a week would work, Ellen decided, and she and the doctor worked out a plan so that she could have the cookies, increasing her predinner dose of Regular insulin twice a week. Ellen left feeling less angry and more in control, and considerably less overwhelmed by her disease.

PHYSICAL ACTIVITY

Everyone, not just children and teenagers with diabetes, should get regular exercise. Exercise is important for general physical fitness and health. It keeps the body in better shape and helps to normalize blood lipids. Individuals who are physically fit are more sensitive to insulin, and this allows them to use lower doses.

However, for the child or teen with diabetes, exercise is not only a beneficial activity but also a factor that must be weighed in calculations about insulin doses. The primary risk of exercise is hypoglycemia. Low blood glucose levels can occur immediately after exercise, or in a delayed pattern. Another risk is that if a patient exercises when his blood glucose is high, particularly if there are ketones in the urine, exercise can release stress hormones, actually causing blood glucose to become even higher. This occurrence is relatively uncommon. As the following cases show, an extra level of management is necessary for children and teens who are actively involved in athletics.

CASE STUDY. Neil R. is 16 years old and has had diabetes for 8 years. Throughout high school he was a competitive ice hockey player. Every morning before school he practiced at the ice rink near his home from 5 to 7 A.M. Through careful monitoring, Neil figured out that 8 ounces per hour of non-diet sodas or fruit juice (containing 100 calories, and 25 g of carbohydrate) held his blood glucose level in the target range during the vigorous exercise required during practice. At 7:30 A.M., when practice was over, Neil showered, checked his blood glucose, took his morning insulin dose, ate breakfast, and went to school.

CASE STUDY. Robin S. is 13 years old and has had diabetes for 2 years. She plays basketball three evenings a week and on Saturday afternoons. After her evening games, she noted a drop in her overnight blood glucose levels. In response, she changed her regimen in two ways. On the nights of the evening games, she decreased her evening NPH dose by 20 percent. Before going to bed, she also ate a complex snack that included protein, fat, and carbohydrates. This plan eliminated the overnight lows.

COMPLICATIONS

Families learning the survival skills for managing diabetes must know how to guard against and recognize acute complications and be aware of the risks of chronic complications. Planned daily telephone contact between the family and the health care provider can decrease or eliminate the need for urgent phone calls from the newly diagnosed patient's family. In these early stages of education and management, attention will primarily be focused on the signs and symptoms of the most common acute complications—hypoglycemia, hyperglycemia, ketosis, and diabetic ketoacidosis.

In the case of hypoglycemia, the basic principle is to always have sugar on hand for treatment, and glucagon for severe cases. (Glucagon is a hormone that, when given by injection, causes the release of stored glucose [glycogen] from the liver and raises blood glucose.) Families must also learn the symptoms of hyperglycemia, and when and how it should be treated; and must learn how to monitor urine ketones, what they mean, and what to do when they are positive. These topics are discussed in detail in chapter 10.

Although patients' and families' questions should be answered honestly, we prefer not to dwell on all the details about the chronic, long-term complications of diabetes in the first days and weeks of diabetes management. As patients and families are adjusting to the diagnosis and the changes to their lifestyle which it requires, details about conditions such as blindness, heart disease, and kidney failure are likely only to frighten them and may cause them to lose hope. However, it is better for them to learn about these possibilities from the health care professional than from the media or poorly informed friends or relatives. It is often useful to ask families what they may have heard about diabetes complications, and to use that information as a starting point for education.

Questions about chronic complications can be handled in a positive, upbeat way by emphasizing that their risk can be significantly decreased. Solid scientific data from the Diabetes Control and Complications Trial show conclusively that tighter blood glucose control achieved by intensive management lowers the risk of long-term complications. This does not mean that clinicians should use scare tactics, but the knowledge of risks can be a powerful incentive for taking responsibility for good control. For instance, the knowledge that poor diabetes control carries a risk of impotence and poor growth may give adolescent boys the motivation they need for compliance.

Primary care and specialty clinicians should also emphasize that they are available to help if any complications should develop. It is important that families understand that monitoring for complications is part of good diabetes care and that early interventions are very successful in slowing the progression of complications if they do occur. (See chapter 10 for a more complete discussion of complications of Type 1 diabetes.) Risks cannot be eliminated, but good control means risk reduction. A useful analogy for families is the risk of an automobile accident when drinking. The sober person has a much lower risk of being in an accident than does the person who has been drinking, but there is still a risk. The person in control of diabetes has a much lower risk of developing complications than does a person with little control.

4

Well-Child Care and the Next Steps in Diabetes Management

A s has been emphasized throughout this book, diabetes is largely a disease of home management. But clinicians must anticipate and respond to a number of complex issues that are beyond the capabilities of most families. These issues are described in this chapter, as is the Diabetes Control and Complications Trial, which provides the clinician with valuable management guidelines and rationales for treatment.

Like any other children or adolescents, children with Type 1 diabetes require general health care and should be enrolled in a primary care practice to receive care independent of or parallel to their diabetes coverage. This should include immunizations, routine laboratory monitoring, growth monitoring, health maintenance issues, developmental issues, and preventive care. It is important not to allow the demands of diabetes control and management to cause neglect of the other medical needs of growing children.

The health care provided to children with diabetes should meet all American Academy of Pediatrics recommendations for preventive pediatric health care.

These recommendations include

> growth monitoring;
> blood pressure monitoring;
> vision and hearing screening;
> developmental behavioral screening;
> physical examinations;
> immunizations;
> lead screening;
> hemoglobin and hematocrit;
> urinalysis;
> anticipatory guidance;
> dental referrals;
> cholesterol screening;
> sexually-transmitted-disease screening for sexually active adolescents; and
> tuberculin testing.

Some clinicians find it helpful to create a diabetes-specific flow chart for the child, coordinating diabetes issues with other health and development issues. Six general goals of long-term diabetes management for children and adolescents can be listed:

> normal physical development, with normal height and weight gain and normal timing of adolescent sexual maturation (puberty);
> maintenance of near-normal glucose and glycohemoglobin levels and elimination of all the symptoms of poorly controlled diabetes (i.e., polyuria, polydipsia, nocturia);
> normal weight maintenance, including prevention of obesity and prevention of eating disorders;
> prevention of acute complications, including diabetic ketoacidosis and significant hypoglycemia;
> prevention of long-term complications; and
> prevention of emotional and/or psychosocial problems.

PHYSICAL DEVELOPMENT

One of the primary goals in treating children and teens with diabetes is to help them maintain normal physical growth. This includes normal growth in height and weight, and normal timing of the onset and progression of puberty. Children who are chronically undertreated with insulin will often have poor weight and height gain, delayed skeletal maturation, and delayed puberty. Conversely, children who are overtreated with insulin may gain weight at an excessive rate.

Weight can be a particularly difficult issue. Because insulin is an anabolic hormone, it works to store calories. Without sufficient insulin, individuals not only will be unable to store calories but will lose their own body stores. With too much insulin, individuals will need to overeat to prevent hypoglycemia, thus causing excessive weight gain.

At every visit with the clinician—usually every 3 months for the child or adolescent with diabetes—height and weight should be measured and plotted on standard growth curves so that any variations from normal velocities can be noted and problems with management can be addressed as early as possible.

Ted H.'s growth curve (fig. 4.1) and case study illustrate the impact that undertreatment or inadequate insulin dosages can have on a child's growth.

CASE STUDY. Ted H. was diagnosed with diabetes at age 6; at that time, his height and weight were in the 5th percentile for his age. We did not see him until he was 16 years old, and he had had no medical care at all between the ages of 13 and 16. His mother had been unemployed and had no medical insurance during those years. At 16, Ted was referred to our clinic by the county health department when his mother took him there for medical services. He was 143 centimeters (4 ft, 8 in.) tall, the average height of an 11-year-old boy, and weighed 29 kilograms (63 lb), and his height and weight were both far below the 5th percentile. He was in early puberty. His insulin dose was 13 units of NPH and 2 units of Regular in the morning; and 10 units of NPH and 2 units of Regular in the evening. It was adjusted according to how he felt and how he looked to his mother, with no home blood glucose monitoring.

Ted's glycohemoglobin was 18.2 percent; his thyroid function was normal; his bone age was 13 years, 4 months. His blood glucose was 500 mg/dL and his cholesterol 271 mg/dL. His urine was positive for ketones and glucose, and his electrolytes were normal. He was not in DKA. We admitted him to the hospital for education and regulation.

Ted's control improved significantly and, as his growth chart (fig. 4.1) illustrates, his growth pattern changed dramatically when he was put on appropriate insulin doses. However, his compliance with monitoring re-

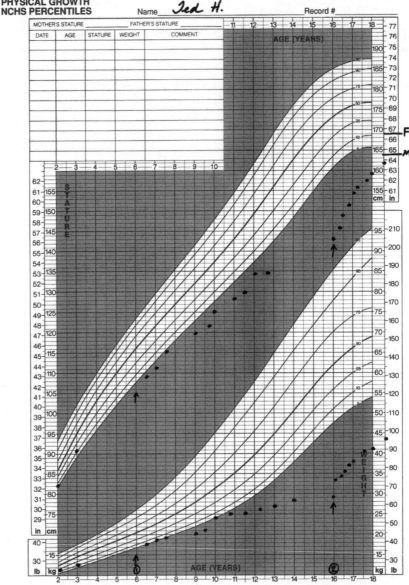

Fig. 4.1. *Solid curves* are growth curves (stature and weight) for various percentiles. *Dotted curves* are Ted H.'s growth curves: *1*, diagnosis of Type 1 diabetes; *2*, first appointment with diabetes clinic, *F*, father's stature; *M*, mother's stature.

The chart showing percentile curves is © 1982 Ross Products Division, Abbott Laboratories. Reprinted by permission. Adapted from P.V.V. Hamill, T. A. Drizd, C. L. Johnson, R. B. Reed, A. F. Roche, and W. M. Moore, "Physical Growth: National Center for Health Statistics Percentiles," American Journal of Clinical Nutrition 32:607–629, 1979. Data from the National Center for Health Statistics (NCHS), Hyattsville, Maryland.

mained intermittent. By the time he was 18, his height was 165 centimeters (65 in.) and his weight was 55 kilograms (120 lb), back up to the 5th percentile for his age.

In contrast, with good long-term control the growth of a child with diabetes can be totally normal, as figure 4.2 shows. This is the growth curve for Amy M., who was profiled in the Introduction.

MEASURING GLYCOHEMOGLOBIN LEVELS

Meticulous blood glucose monitoring is the cornerstone and the framework of good diabetes management, essential to the development of an understanding of the dynamics of this disease. Daily self-monitoring of blood glucose is the responsibility of children and teenagers with diabetes and their families, a survival skill that they must be taught in the first days following diagnosis (see chapter 3). The measurement of glycohemoglobin is the responsibility of the health care provider.

One of the most important advances in diabetes management in the past two decades has been the discovery of and the ability to reliably measure glycohemoglobin—also called glycosylated hemoglobin or glycated hemoglobin—or its fractions, hemoglobin A_1 (HbA$_1$) and hemoglobin A_{1C} (HbA$_{1C}$). Glycohemoglobin is an objective measure of the individual patient's average blood glucose control over the 2- to 3-month period before the level is determined. It is objective because it does not depend on the accuracy, frequency, or timing of the patient's blood glucose monitoring and recording. Other glycosylated proteins, specifically fructosamine and glycated albumin, are not as useful in long-term diabetes management and are not frequently used clinically.

Glycohemoglobin is formed by an irreversible attachment of glucose molecules to free amino groups in the hemoglobin molecule. This attachment is proportional to the blood glucose concentration—that is, the higher the blood glucose, the more glucose attaches to hemoglobin, and the more glycohemoglobin is formed. Glycohemoglobin can be measured at any time of day and is not affected by the blood glucose concentration at the time of sampling.

Glycohemoglobin can be measured on a venipuncture specimen or a capillary sample, depending on the method used by each specific laboratory. There are a number of assay methods. Normal ranges vary depending

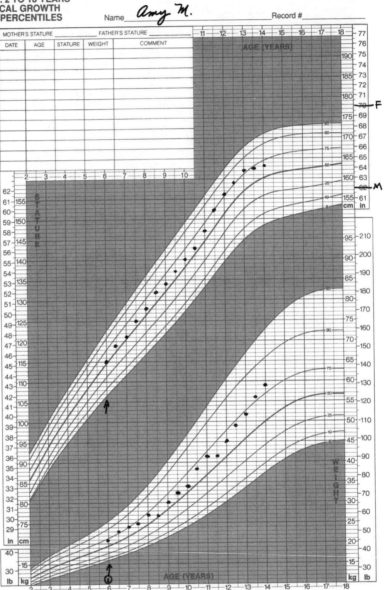

Fig. 4.2. *Solid curves* are growth curves (stature and weight) for various percentiles. *Dotted curves* are the growth curves for Amy M., a girl with diabetes with a normal growth pattern: *I*, diagnosis of Type 1 diabetes; *F*, father's stature; *M*, mother's stature.

on the assay used, and it is not possible to compare results obtained by different assays and different laboratories. It is important for each clinician to know the method used in each laboratory he or she uses, the normal range for that assay, and what confounding factors can interfere with the assay.

Of the several assay methods used to measure glycohemoglobin, some are affected by hemoglobinopathy or anemia; some measure only HbA_{1C}; and some measure other glycohemoglobin subfractions. The assays used are high performance liquid chromatography (HPLC), ion exchange chromatography, affinity chromatography, immunoassays, electrophoresis, and colorimetric assays.

In sum, the important points for the primary care clinician to remember are that it is essential to know your laboratory's glycohemoglobin assay and the assay's normal (non-diabetic) range, and that one must keep in mind that some assays are affected by hemoglobinopathies.

Unfortunately, there is no standardization across the United States in measuring glycohemoglobin levels. Comparing glycohemoglobin levels from different assays is comparing apples and oranges. Families might find this difficult to understand, and when presenting glycohemoglobin results to families, it is important to always put them in the context of normal (nondiabetic) ranges.

It is also important for the clinician to compare the patient's glycohemoglobin level to reported blood glucose levels obtained from self-monitoring. Discrepancies may indicate either inaccurate or fabricated blood glucose measurements or determinations that are so infrequent that average blood glucose levels are not adequately represented. For example, one 16-year-old boy told us that he does not check his blood glucose when he knows it is high, because it ruins the running average in his meter. Other children and teens may check but not record a high blood glucose level to avoid unpleasant confrontations with their parents.

Glycohemoglobin measurements help the clinician, the patient, and the family to plan and to adjust their goals. They help them assess how changes in their therapeutic regimen are working and to determine when extra help and attention are needed. Measuring glycohemoglobin levels every 3 months is usually recommended in children and teens with diabetes. However, during periods of intensification of control (i.e., when the child is beginning to use an insulin pump or multiple daily injections) or when the regimen is changed for other reasons (e.g., a new sports schedule), more frequent measurements to assess the trend in glycohemoglobins may help to evaluate how the new regimen is working.

We generally recommend that the glycohemoglobin goal for older children and teens be similar to the glycohemoglobin in the DCCT intensive control group: about 1 to 1.5 percent above the upper limit of normal for that assay. In younger (i.e., preschool) children, acceptable levels are a bit higher because of the difficulties that young children may have in detecting early signs of low blood glucose and communicating symptoms to their parents or caretakers. Also, younger children are likely to be more irregular eaters than older children, which puts them more at risk for hypoglycemia. Table 4.1 lists the various assays.

MONITORING FOR COMPLICATIONS

Most of the long-term complications of diabetes are caused by chronic hyperglycemia and will be discussed below. The most acute problem associated with hyperglycemia is diabetic ketoacidosis, and a major goal of diabetes management is to avoid DKA. This can be done by monitoring urine for ketones, which are the first sign of ketoacidosis. Ketones appear in the urine when body fats are broken down for energy, an indication that there is insufficient insulin for normal metabolism.

Ketones can be present for days before a person becomes acidotic. The urine of a child or adolescent with diabetes should be checked for ketones whenever the child is sick in any way, but particularly when she is sick with stomach aches, nausea, vomiting, diarrhea, or fever, or whenever the blood glucose level is high (usually defined as greater than 250 or 300 mg/dL). Vomiting can be both a sign of early ketoacidosis and a symptom that can push a person into ketoacidosis. Patients and families can check for urine ketones at home with an inexpensive commercially available dipstick test.

Monitoring for long-term complications of diabetes is important. The earliest sign of nephropathy is the spilling of small amounts of albumin in the urine. While urine dipsticks to check for protein are easily available, they measure only relatively high levels of protein. There are newer, more sensitive methods to detect microalbumin, tiny amounts of protein that the dipsticks are not sensitive enough to pick up. Most medical centers monitor microalbumin annually in children and teenagers with diabetes (see chapter 10).

Blood pressure should also be measured at least annually. Blood pressure above the 90th percentile for the child's age is a cause for concern and may require intervention. Hypertension is a significant risk factor for dia-

Table 4.1.   **Summary of Methods for Determination of Glycated Hemoglobin**

Method[a]	Assay Type	Component Measured	Assay Interference by	
			Hemoglobin-opathy	Nonglucose Adducts
Affinity chromatography				
Glyc-Affin (Isolab)	AC minicolumn	GHb	No	No
GlycoTest (Pierce)	AC minicolumn	GHb	No	No
Glyco-Tek (Helena)	AC minicolumn	GHb	No	No
Vision GHb (Abbott)	AC column	GHb	No	No
IMx$_{1c}$ (Abbott)	AC	GHb	No	No
CLC330 (Primus)	Affinity HPLC	GHb	No	No
Merck HPLC (Merck)	Affinity HPLC	GHb	No	No
Ion-exchange chromatography				
Quik-Sep (Isolab)	IEC minicolumn	HbA$_1$	Yes	Yes
HbA$_{1c}$ column (Bio-Rad)	IEC minicolumn	HbA$_{1c}$	Yes	Yes
Glyco Hb Quik (Helena)	IEC minicolumn	HbA$_1$	Yes	Yes
Diamat (Bio-Rad)	HPLC	HbA$_{1c}$	Yes	Yes
Variant (Bio-Rad)	HPLC	HbA$_{1c}$	Yes	Yes
Modular (Bio-Rad)	HPLC	HbA$_{1c}$	Yes	Yes
Pharmacia	HPLC	HbA$_{1c}$	Yes	Yes
Menarini	HPLC	HbA$_{1c}$	Yes	Yes
Watres	HPLC	HbA$_{1c}$	Yes	Yes
Biomen	HPLC	HbA$_{1c}$	Yes	Yes
Vydac	HPLC	HbA$_{1c}$	Yes	Yes
Immunoassay				
DCA 2000 (Miles)	Immunoassay	HbA$_{1c}$	No	No
Dako test (Novoclone)	Immunoassay	HbA$_{1c}$	Yes	No
Hemoglobin A1c Tina-quant (Boehringer Mannheim)	Immunoassay	HbA$_{1c}$	No	No
Electrophoresis				
Glytrak (Corning)	Electrophoresis	HbA$_1$	Yes	Yes
REP Glyco-30 (Helena)	Electrophoresis	HbA$_1$	Yes	Yes
Diatrac HbA$_{1c}$ (Helena)	Electrophoresis	HbA$_{1c}$	Yes	Yes
Colorimetric				
Thiobarbituric acid	Colorimetric	GHb	No	No

Source: Adapted, with permission, from American Diabetes Association, *Intensive Diabetes Management* (Alexandria, Va.: ADA, 1993), 85.

Note: This table may not include all of the available tests. Some tests are in widespread usage; others are used less frequently.

[a]*Abbreviations*: AC, affinity chromatography; GHb, glycohemoglobin; HbA$_1$, hemoglobin A$_1$; HbA$_{1c}$, hemoglobin A$_{1c}$; IEC, ion exchange chromatography.

betic nephropathy and is also of concern because people with diabetes are also at higher risk for macrovascular diseases. Blood lipids should also be monitored after diagnosis, with a breakdown including total cholesterol, high-density lipoprotein (HDL), low-density lipoprotein (LDL), and triglycerides. If the results are normal, repeat measurements should be obtained every 5 years. If they are abnormal, more frequent monitoring is necessary.

Children and adolescents with diabetes should also be monitored with annual ophthalmologic examinations, which should begin 3 to 5 years after diagnosis. Screening is usually not needed before 10 years of age, unless there is some indication of vision problems or abnormalities.

Clinicians treating children with diabetes should have an awareness of associated autoimmune diseases, particularly thyroid abnormalities. As many as 20 percent of persons with Type 1 diabetes may have thyroid autoimmunity. In our clinic, we monitor with testing for thyroid-stimulating hormone (TSH) and thyroid antibodies and look for clinical signs of abnormal thyroid function. This is usually done shortly after a diabetes diagnosis and every few years thereafter. If there are any suspicious signs, we will check more frequently for thyroid abnormality. In children with diabetes, poor linear growth can be attributed to both poor diabetes control and the development of another autoimmune endocrine disease, particularly hypothyroidism.

Clinicians treating children with diabetes should also have a heightened awareness of the potential for psychological, social, and behavioral problems in these patients. Attentiveness to these issues can lead to early intervention and referral to a mental health professional. Psychological issues are discussed more fully in chapter 11.

Another important concern that is sometimes overlooked is the necessity for seasonal adjustments for many children and teens with diabetes. Families and clinicians need to be aware that the changing seasons can bring lifestyle changes that need to be taken into account in the regimen of the child with diabetes. For the majority of children, as spring arrives and warmer weather prevails, and especially as the school year ends, physical activity increases, sometimes markedly. This leads to increased risk of mild, moderate, or severe hypoglycemia (depending on the level of activity) and necessitates a change in the therapeutic regimen, with increases in caloric intake, decreases in insulin dosage, or both. Attendance at summer camp, with increased physical activity, may also increase the risk of hypoglycemia.

Conversely, when summer ends and school begins, the decreased physical activity may lead to an increased risk of hyperglycemia, necessitating a regimen change with reduced calories, increased insulin, or both.

MAINTENANCE OF NORMAL WEIGHT

The daily management of dietary issues falls to the family, not the clinician, and is covered in several other sections of this book. Dietary needs are constantly changing in growing children and teens. Calories and nutrients need to be assessed in an ongoing manner and adjusted as needed for a growing child or teen. One of the most important things to remember about modern management of diabetes is that there are no longer forbidden foods. Again, sugar does not have to be avoided—although it must be covered with the appropriate amount of insulin. Like everyone else, children or teens with diabetes should eat a prudent, low-fat, high-fiber diet. They should be aware that sugar comes from many sources; the body does not care if it came from a cookie or a potato: it is still glucose, with the same metabolic demands.

Monitoring weight at every clinic visit, just like monitoring height, is important for early detection of deviations from normal patterns.

IMMUNIZATIONS

Children and teenagers with diabetes should receive all immunizations as recommended by the American Academy of Pediatrics (AAP), and they should receive them at the standard ages. As new vaccines are developed, primary care clinicians should follow AAP recommendations for their patients with diabetes, as well as for their patients without diabetes.

Influenza vaccines are recommended for people with chronic diseases, including diabetes. Families should be aware of these recommendations. However, it is not clear that healthy children and teenagers with diabetes are any more susceptible to influenza than are any other children. It is also important that families understand that the vaccines prevent only the types of influenza covered by that specific vaccine. Influenza vaccines do *not* protect against any other viruses that cause respiratory infections or gastroenteritis. Children and teens with diabetes have their most significant management problems when illnesses with vomiting occur, and there are no vaccines currently available to prevent these. Therefore, we think that the decision about whether or not to vaccinate a child with diabetes against influenza should be left up to the individual family, as long as they understand these issues.

THE DIABETES CONTROL AND COMPLICATIONS TRIAL AND ITS IMPLICATIONS FOR MEDICAL MANAGEMENT

The Diabetes Control and Complications Trial was a 10-year, multicenter, randomized trial that compared the effects of intensive and conventional Type 1 diabetes management on long-term diabetes complications. The results of the trial—first announced in 1993—confirmed that good day-to-day management pays off in the long term. Control matters. These findings have important implications for clinicians treating patients with Type 1 diabetes.

More than 1,400 patients, aged 13 to 39, were randomized into two groups:

➤ Members of the intensive therapy group took three or more insulin injections a day or used continuous subcutaneous insulin infusion through a pump. They monitored blood glucose levels at least four times a day and adjusted insulin doses accordingly. They had monthly appointments and even more frequent telephone contact with the study center. Their glycohemoglobin levels were measured every month.

➤ Members of the conventional therapy group took one or two injections of insulin daily. They monitored their blood (or urine) glucose levels once a day and had medical appointments and glycohemoglobin measures every 3 months.

One focus of the study was the development or progression of retinopathy, a significant risk in patients with Type 1 diabetes. In the intensive therapy group, the development of retinopathy was reduced by 76 percent in patients who did not already have it, and progression of this complication was reduced by 54 percent in patients who already had it. Analyses showed a steadily increasing risk of retinopathy progression with increasing mean glycohemoglobin levels. Similar significant findings were observed in the onset and progression of nephropathy and neuropathy. In other words, the lower glycemic levels achieved by intensive management delay the onset and slow the progression of the most serious medical complications associated with Type 1 diabetes.

An important message of the DCCT concerns the incremental association of glycemic control and the development or progression of complications. For each decrement in glycohemoglobin, there is an associated decrease in the risk of complications. Therefore, any improvement in glycemic control is helpful. Decreases do not have to be dramatic for positive outcomes to occur.

However, a risk of intensive management was also identified in the DCCT. There was a threefold increase in severe hypoglycemic episodes (defined as episodes requiring assistance from another person) in the intensive management group. Intensive control was also associated with weight gain.

Something else that the DCCT made clear was that adolescents—who accounted for 195 of the patients in the trial—are more difficult to manage than adult patients and require a greater proportion of the resources of the management team. This comes as no surprise to clinicians with experience in caring for adolescents with chronic disease.

The application of DCCT results to younger children is not so definitive. Children under the age of 13 years were not studied in this trial. In very young children, risk-to-benefit ratios for intensive management are less likely to be favorable. Because the risks of hypoglycemia are high in young children and may have more serious negative effects on brain development and long-term cognitive function, the blood glucose and glycohemoglobin goals of the DCCT are not reasonable for children under the age of 7 years. As a rough guideline, aiming for HbA_{1C} levels in the low 7's (i.e., 7.2%, which was the DCCT mean for the adult intensive management group; normal range < 6.05%) or even 8's may put many children below the age of 4 to 5 at high risk for severe hypoglycemia. For children between 5 and 7, especially if the child is able to recognize and communicate hypoglycemic symptoms, tighter control might be considered. Clearly, families need to know the DCCT data, understand the benefits and risks of improved glycemic control, and decide, with their clinicians, what level of control is reasonable for their children at different ages.

5

Educating Patients and Families

with Loretta Clark, R.N., C.D.E.

As emphasized in a number of different contexts above, education of patients and their families is a fundamental component of successful diabetes management. This education must be ongoing, and it must be comprehensive. From the time of diagnosis, all but the youngest children need to know something about what causes diabetes and what it will mean to their lives. As they grow older they will be able to handle increasingly sophisticated explanations. Many children with diabetes and their families become as knowledgeable about this condition as their health care providers, and sometimes more so.

In the beginning, though, many people may harbor misinformation and skewed perceptions. Families may get inaccurate information from older relatives who did not have the benefit of modern diabetes management. A child may know of a relative who had diabetes-related complications and may be terrified of the disease. Another, who knows a peer who deals with the demands of diabetes without much apparent disruption to her life, may seem less threatened. It's always important to ask parents and older children what their preconceptions are, what they already know (or think they know) about diabetes, so that they will not continue to harbor false notions.

One of the most difficult concepts to accept about diabetes is that it is a lifelong disease. We have found that parents and children receive this information with varying reactions. You will see sadness, anger, and fear. They may mourn the passing of "normal" family life. It is not uncommon to encounter regret and grief on the part of parents who think that their perfect child is no longer perfect. Children sometimes want to express their anger by striking out, by hitting. It can be very therapeutic for them to direct their anger at a punching bag, or a pillow with a sign on it that says "diabetes." Guilt and denial are also typical reactions. Children will feel guilty for bringing this burden to the family; parents will feel guilty for having somehow caused the disease in their child.

The diagnosis of diabetes will draw these families into a new world, with different rules and a new framework for their lives. Diabetes has its own language: *highs* and *lows* (referring to blood glucose levels), *drawing up* (insulin into the syringe), *falling out* (passing out from low blood sugar), *bottoming out* (a hospital term for low blood glucose), and *downloading the meter*, to name just a few commonly used terms. This can sometimes lead to confusion, although it can also be amusing:

> CASE STUDY.   Johnny M. is 13 years old, has good control, and manages his diabetes well. He is open in talking with his friends about life with diabetes. One afternoon his mother received a phone call at home from a substitute teacher at Johnny's school. Obviously feeling that she was dealing with a very sensitive issue, the teacher spoke in a whisper. "Mrs. M., I'm afraid that Johnny may be using drugs," she confided. "He said this afternoon that he was feeling high."
>
> "Oh, he's talking about his blood sugar," said Mrs. M., laughing. "He has diabetes."

WHAT TO TEACH, AND WHEN

There is an enormous amount of information associated with diabetes. It is important not to overload families and patients with more than they can handle in the days immediately following diagnosis. This does not mean that all of their questions shouldn't be answered honestly. But some topics are better deferred for a later time when they feel more confident of their ability to live with diabetes and are beginning to master some of the skills necessary for diabetes management.

We recommend educating patients from the start of the hospitalization period. Indeed, as noted above, newly diagnosed diabetes patients are sometimes hospitalized not only for medical reasons but also to make the patient and family available for the intense barrage of information they will need to assimilate. The first task is to introduce them to the basic survival skills (see chapter 3). However, it is important for the clinician to be aware that at this stressful time many people will not remember all the details and particulars that are presented to them. We tell them not to worry about remembering everything, that we will be available for continuing referral and consultation, and that there are a number of publications available for reference. We also give our patients a reference book or two that they can keep. We like *Understanding Insulin-Dependent Diabetes Mellitus* (known as the "Pink Panther" book), by Peter Chase, and *An Instructional Aid on Insulin-Dependent Diabetes Mellitus*, by Luther Travis.

During the initial hospitalization, someone from our team—usually the nurse educator—talks with patients and their families daily in an educational session. We explain the tasks that are being performed for daily management—specifically, adjustment of insulin doses and review of the actual blood glucose measurements. We are very specific about what is being done, and why. For example, we will tell a patient and his family, "Your before-dinner blood sugar is elevated, so we'll increase the morning dose of NPH to bring it down." We make it clear why we are making the adjustments that we are making, and we begin to introduce the basic guidelines that will help them to make these decisions on their own.

At the patient's first follow-up visit, usually 2 weeks after diagnosis, we review injection and blood glucose monitoring techniques. It is important to emphasize from the beginning of the educational process that diabetes is a self-management disease and that the eventual goal is for us to serve as consultants. A clinician actually observes how the patient (or parent) draws up, injects, and does the monitoring. Patients need to master the particulars of whatever meter they are using to monitor blood glucose. We teach them how to check the meter for accuracy, using check strips and a glucose control solution. Some meters require cleaning. All of these tasks are done according to the manufacturer's recommendations, which come with the meter. There are approximately 20 different meters on the market, and the American Diabetes Association publishes a useful guide to them. We find that with the pediatric population, it is helpful to have a meter that remembers not just the blood glucose level but also the date and time of the sample and has the capability for computer hookup to graph and print out the data.

Although patients and their parents need to understand that there are serious short- and long-term consequences of poorly managed diabetes, diabetes educators should avoid using scare tactics or worst-case scenarios. However, it is important that families and older children understand that they are in charge of their health and that the actions they take now will have long-term consequences.

By the end of the initial education period, the clinician should be clear that the patient (if he is old enough) and his family understand the following concepts:

> Diabetes is a disease of insulin deficiency.
> Insulin-dependent diabetes is the result of an autoimmune process in which the body has killed off the insulin-producing beta cells.
> It is a lifelong condition. Once the beta cells are gone, they cannot be restored or replaced by current medical technology.
> Insulin is needed for the cells to obtain normal nourishment. A person cannot live without insulin.
> Diabetes is treated by providing insulin by injection a minimum of twice a day.
> The treatment is imperfect because with current replacement techniques it is not possible to accurately mimic pancreatic insulin production.

Appendix D shows a questionnaire that we give to patients or to families of patients who have been diagnosed elsewhere and are coming to us for the first time. Appendix E shows our patient education plan, with spaces for documentation. Also see chapter 3.

OVERCOMING FEARS

One of the most important purposes of diabetes education is to help people overcome their fears. It is usually helpful to confront these fears early in the education process and get them out of the way. This head-on approach can serve to alleviate anxieties about many issues that the family is facing.

Through the years, we have seen that in diabetes management, considerable fear—on the part of both children and parents—often centers around the actual injections. Many people are afraid of needles. People fear the pain of injection, and they are afraid that they could cause harm with improper technique. When teaching patients and families how to give injections, it is useful to give normal saline injections to the parents so that they will experience just what their child is feeling. The pain is minimal, a tiny pinprick. When thinking of needles, many people think of the burning of penicillin injections, with the long needle required for intramuscular injections. However, the ultrafine needles now used for insulin injections—which are subcutaneous—cause little pain (see fig. 6.1).

Many children also have problems with the pain of the finger-stick for blood glucose monitoring. Distraction—for instance, letting them watch a favorite video during the stick or injection—often works well for younger children. Allowing the child to make choices also helps. Let her choose which finger to prick for the blood glucose check, and which site to use for the insulin injection.

Parents should take a positive attitude in approaching these tasks with their child. If parents have negative feelings about giving their child injections or finger-pricks, these feelings will inevitably be transferred to the child, to some extent. A parent's comment that "I know this hurts" or "I wish I didn't have to do this" can only make a child more fearful and apprehensive. Instead, parents should take a more positive approach with comments such as "This hurts a little, but the hurt will stop in a few seconds," or "You're being very helpful by holding so still."

> CASE STUDY.   Anna L. is 7 years old and hates getting her insulin injections. During a clinic visit, her parents revealed that they sometimes spent 90 minutes negotiating with Anna before the shot was given, as Anna's father tried to persuade her that she was ready, and waited for the child to agree. Meanwhile, Anna would be crying and pleading, "Wait, wait, please wait."
>
> Anna's mother is more direct in her approach. She will say, "This has to be done and I'm going to do it now." This makes the mother the "heavy," and Anna tries to get her father to give her the injections.

This illustrates that there are some choices that children should not have. They must know that there is no choice about getting injections or about monitoring; that these procedures will be performed is a given, and they must be done within a reasonable period of time. Parents can be firm without being mean. Sometimes—most often in the case of children under the age of 7—the task of giving injections will take both parents: one to keep the child still, the other to give the shot. Some approaches are more effective than others. Rather than saying, "I have to hold you down," a father might say, "I'm going to help you calm down and get comfortable while Mommy gives you the shot." Generally, physical resistance will not continue for long. If the child is still upset after the shot, parents should be calm and comforting and give reinforcement: "You really held still today, Anna, and that helped me a lot with the injection."

What finally turned the corner for Anna was when her parents allowed her to give her own shots. They drew up the insulin and the child injected it. We cautioned the family, though, that a child of this age needs to be carefully supervised to ensure that the injection is providing the proper dose and that insulin is not leaking out when the shot is given. Parents of children of this age should also understand that the child may want to assume a certain task but may soon lose interest. Children shouldn't be forced to take on a responsibility for which they are not ready.

Babies will not have the same fear of needles as young children, but sometimes their constant activity can make it very difficult to give a shot. A parent can handle a wriggly baby alone by clamping the baby's feet between her legs, wrapping one arm around the baby to hold the upper body still, and using her other arm to give the shot. In taking blood from a baby for a glucose check, some parents find it easier to use a pipette or glass capillary tube to withdraw the blood and then transfer it to the blood glucose strip for the meter, rather than trying to capture blood directly on the strip.

Another common fear of parents is that they will inadvertently do something to hurt their child. Fears sometimes center around the use of glucagon and the possibility that they might overtreat their child. In fact, there is no significant risk from a glucagon injection.

We find that most parents (and grandparents, in some cases) become comfortable with giving injections after only a few days. Usually the job of giving injections becomes the routine task of one parent. We encourage the other parent to become involved in other ways—for instance, by purchasing supplies and charting blood glucose levels.

If children are doing the injections themselves, there are specific aids that can help if they have a needle phobia. Sometimes simply seeing the syringe and the needle scares them. A product called Inject-ease is a slip-cover-like hard plastic sheath that masks the needle so that the child can't see it. If a needle phobia persists despite the parents' best efforts to work the child through it, professional psychological counseling may help to identify the underlying fears.

In the past, we would teach our patients to pull back the plunger and check for blood coming back into the syringe to make sure that they hadn't hit a major blood vessel. That is no longer the practice for subcutaneous injections, because with the tiny needles that are used today, the chances of this happening are minimal.

Sometimes a clinician will see a child who does extremely well with injections in the beginning but 3 to 6 months later begins to develop a phobia. It is difficult to know for sure why this happens, but it may be related to a particularly painful injection or to blood leakage.

THE FINE POINTS OF BLOOD GLUCOSE MONITORING

CASE STUDY.   Derrick M. is 6 years old, and he knows just what to do when he gets a cut on his finger. He runs to get his glucose meter and lets his bleeding finger drip onto the strip. "Why let that good blood go down the drain?" he reasons.

Parents who are having difficulty getting the drop of blood necessary for blood glucose monitoring can improve their technique by following a few simple guidelines. For best results, they should get a good hanging drop of blood before trying to apply it to the monitor strip. If they are having trouble, they may not be applying sufficient pressure. If the child has a tendency to move his finger, it may be easier to keep him still if they place his hand on a table. Washing the child's hands in warm water prior to the procedure can help increase circulation to the fingertips, as can windmilling the arm, shaking the hand down, and keeping the hand below the level of the heart. Another technique is to "milk" the finger, pressing out a drop of blood.

Children who are having trouble with monitoring may think that they have more control if they choose the finger to be pricked. To avoid scarring and calluses, however, it is important not always to use the same finger for the prick. There is a better blood supply on the side of the fingertip than in the middle. Also, the middle of the fingertip is more sensitive and may hurt more.

Children should be taught not to lick their finger after the prick, because there are bacteria in the mouth that could cause an infection. It is necessary to wash hands before the finger-stick to decrease the chance of infection and to remove food and drink residue from the finger. However, it is not necessary to wipe the finger with alcohol, although many people choose to do this. Children and teens doing self-monitoring of blood glucose should also be aware that it is easy for the sample to become contaminated. For example, if the child was eating an apple and there is juice from the apple on the finger, this can affect the reading.

Parents are often concerned about overnight or early-morning lows, and blood glucose monitoring is sometimes necessary during the night, particularly as routines are being established and dosages determined. During this period, it is usually a good idea to do routine checks between 2 A.M. and 3 A.M. Often, children do not even awaken for this prick. However, they should know ahead of time that this will be occurring during the night, and they should be given the choice of whether they want to be awakened or not.

Health professionals and parents should avoid using judgmental terms such as *good* or *bad* to refer to blood glucose monitoring results. Results should be described as "high," "low," or "in the target range." Children shouldn't think that an out-of-target count means that they have failed a test, and they should never be punished for a result. This kind of attitude may lead to obfuscation of results. We have seen some creative excuses from children, who will "forget" to bring a meter to a clinic appointment or will take out the batteries to erase the memory. Some children have found that they can trick their meters with red food coloring, fingernail polish, or even a friend's blood.

LEARNING ABOUT GLUCAGON

Glucagon is injected to treat severe insulin reactions when the patient is unconscious, having a seizure, or otherwise unable to eat or drink. Learning how to use glucagon is an important part of the diabetes education process. While patients should be familiar with what glucagon does and how it is used, education about glucagon is primarily directed at parents and siblings, since they will make the decision to use glucagon and will do the injecting.

Glucagon is available in two forms: in two vials (glucagon and diluent) to be drawn up and mixed and then drawn into the syringe; and in a glucagon emergency kit with one vial, with the diluent in the syringe. We recommend the emergency kit, because the diluent is already drawn up in the syringe, saving an extra step. To use it, one injects the diluting solution into the powdered glucagon tablet in the vial, shakes it a couple of times, and draws back the entire amount into the syringe. When injecting glucagon, the skin should not be pinched up as it is for an insulin injection; it should be pulled smooth and the glucagon should be shot straight in, so that the deeper injection can allow faster absorption. The dose is the whole vial (1 mg), except for babies weighing less than 10 kilograms (22 lb), for whom half a vial (0.5 mg) is recommended.

Our philosophy about using glucagon is simple: when in doubt, use it. It won't hurt, and it can quickly remedy a risky situation. Glucagon acts quickly, but not instantaneously—even though the blood glucose does start rising upon injection, it usually takes about 10 minutes for the child to respond. Glucagon is short-acting, and once the child or teen regains consciousness he will need food and/or drink.

Many children and teenagers with diabetes will probably never use glucagon. But it is an important part of the diabetes armamentarium, something that should be kept in the home of every person with diabetes. If there is a nurse at the child's school, glucagon should also be kept in the nurse's office. It should be taken along on vacations and trips, and the expiration date should be checked regularly. When the glucagon is past its expiration date, it is a good idea to practice mixing it and drawing it up (but *not* injecting) before discarding it. This helps parents feel more comfortable if a real emergency arises.

Children and teens with diabetes usually learn to recognize early symptoms of hypoglycemia and alleviate them with some form of oral glucose. However, some people are more prone to hypoglycemic unawareness and can't tell when their blood glucose is dropping, or confuse the symptoms with something else. Continued hypoglycemia over a period of several days can exacerbate the unawareness. Hypoglycemia and hypoglycemic unawareness are discussed more fully in chapter 10.

INTERACTION WITH SCHOOLS

It is important that families of children and adolescents with diabetes have a close and ongoing relationship with the child's school. Because of issues of medical confidentiality, the first notification of the disease must come from the parents, not the health care provider. We recommend that a conference, with parents, teacher(s), and the school nurse present, be arranged as soon as possible after the diagnosis. Other school personnel who need to be educated about diabetes include the principal, school bus drivers, coaches, physical education teachers, substitute teachers, and cafeteria workers. A sample letter for parents to send to school personnel is included in Appendix F. Appendix G is a letter from the physician to the teacher.

There are also videotapes and pamphlets available to teach school personnel about diabetes. The Juvenile Diabetes Foundation and the American Diabetes Association are good sources of such materials. See Appendix I, "Resources," for more suggestions.

It is important that school personnel know that a hypoglycemic reaction needs to be treated immediately and know how to recognize and treat one. A general guideline is: when in doubt, treat. If a child has been treated during the day for a low, the parents should be notified at the end of the school day. The more information parents can give school personnel about the specific symptoms with which their child responds to a low—for example, her legs get wobbly, he gets a fluttery feeling in his stomach, she falls asleep —the more knowledgeable a response school personnel will have. When his blood glucose is running high, a child may have to make frequent trips to the bathroom to urinate, or leave the class for drinks. A child with diabetes should never be allowed to fall asleep in a class.

> CASE STUDY.   Scott P. is 12 years old, a seventh grader. One morning, in a class being taught by a substitute teacher, he fell asleep. He was allowed to sleep for the whole class, which was just prior to his scheduled lunch period. When the period ended, the teacher shook him and was not able to arouse him. Scott had not told anyone that he had been in such a hurry that morning that he had skipped breakfast; this was the reason for his low blood glucose level. The school did not have a school nurse, so there was no glucagon on hand. Scott was taken by ambulance to a local emergency department and was unarousable for several hours, even though his hypoglycemia was quickly corrected.

A child or adolescent with diabetes should never be sent alone to the nurse's office. If the child is feeling low and needs to check a blood glucose level, another responsible student should accompany her to the nurse's office. Ideally, we recommend that symptoms of low blood glucose be treated right in the classroom. It is our experience that many schools will not allow blood glucose monitoring in the classroom.

Because we are aiming for tighter control of blood glucose levels, more children are at risk for hypoglycemia at school. Also, some children may be on a regimen that necessitates getting injections at school. We generally do not recommend injections at school for children younger than about 7 years old, because dose decisions can be complicated and there is potential for error unless a responsible adult can be in charge. Schools require specific written guidelines from physicians for medications to be given at school.

Schoolchildren with diabetes should have a kit of "survival" supplies, which can be contained in a plastic sandwich bag. Such a bag can be provided to each teacher for each classroom. The kit might contain glucose tablets, a fruit drink box, raisins, a tube of cake icing, glucose gel, and peanut butter crackers. There should also be specific instructions related to the individual. For instance: "I have diabetes. I take insulin, and if my blood sugar gets too low, I get shaky, dizzy, headachy, sweaty, sleepy, and hungry. If this happens, give me one-third of a tube of cake icing and call my mother at 555-1234. If there is no improvement in 15 minutes, give me another one-third tube of icing and a peanut butter cracker."

Eating snacks is often not allowed in the classroom, which can present a problem for the child with diabetes. If a child needs to leave the classroom twice a day for snacks, and a third time for monitoring, this could amount to up to an hour a day of missed classroom time. We have seen, in elementary school, how a sensitive and understanding teacher can work the whole class's snack time around the schedule of the child with diabetes, so that he is not set apart from the others by having to leave the class to eat or by eating alone in the classroom.

> CASE STUDY.   Karen A., 10 years old, endured teasing from her cousins and classmates after her diagnosis with diabetes. "You've got diabetes," they would taunt her. Or "I don't want to play with you because you've got diabetes," or "I might catch it."

Any condition that brands a child as different can result in teasing. A sensitivity or diversity training session for the other children in the class can be helpful. A school nurse, a diabetes nurse educator, or even a parent or knowledgeable teacher can run the session. One way to introduce the subject is to talk about differences among children. "Some kids have brown hair, some have black hair, some kids have asthma, some have diabetes." A parent can demonstrate how injections are given and how blood glucose monitoring is done. Children's perceptions can shift after a presentation like this, as they suddenly see their schoolmate not as different but as a brave person who has to have injections every day. However, one should never invade the privacy of the child with diabetes. It is important that the child know about the information that will be presented, and agree to the presentation. Some children are very private about their condition, and the amount of personal detail that is presented should be their choice.

Our diabetes nurse educator was once invited to the birthday party of a 7 year old who had recently been diagnosed with diabetes. She talked to the children about diabetes, showed them insulin and syringes, demonstrated an injection on a doll, and measured the birthday girl's blood glucose before eating birthday cake.

DIABETES IN THE FAMILY

In general we work with families as a unit, with children and teens individually, and with parents individually or in groups. The psychological and emotional issues can often be handled well in a group situation, in which parents can benefit from hearing about how others have dealt with the problems and life changes resulting from diabetes.

Managing diabetes will affect family dynamics and may highlight or intensify problems. In general, some of the most difficult family issues focus on the transfer of responsibility for diabetes management from parent to child. Different children become capable at different ages, and no child should be pushed into these responsibilities until he thinks he is ready for them. This issue is very specific to diabetes; we see some families struggle while others function more smoothly. The transition should be very gradual. If the parent and child work together when the child is younger, and the parent progressively passes on skills and techniques to the child, this will enable a smooth transition.

As children reach mid–elementary school age, they will be able to take on increasing responsibility for managing and understanding their disease. By the age of 9 years, children can usually start to take over insulin injections with the assistance of a parent. Drawing up the insulin is more difficult than actually giving the injection. Sometimes a diabetes camp experience, where a group of peers is giving injections, is a good place to start for the child who is having trouble. However, although young children may become technically adept at some of the skills necessary for diabetes management—such as measuring and injecting insulin, finger-sticking, and using the blood glucose meter—they may be years away from mastery of the cognitive skills underlying these technical tasks.

By the time most children are in their preteen years, we talk with them directly about insulin dose adjustments related to blood glucose values, changes in activity, and food intake. For older children, especially teenagers, we recommend weekly or twice-weekly diabetes family meetings to discuss the rationale for adjustments, and other issues and problems that must be talked about and thought through. The importance of parental supervision cannot be overemphasized. Deteriorating control can result from a transfer of responsibility without deliberation and appropriate supervision. If a transfer of responsibility is attempted before the child is emotionally and cognitively ready, worsening management may be the outcome.

Even if the child seems to be handling all the technical aspects of diabetes management and making competent decisions, parents should remain aware of everything that is done. Just because a child says in January that he wants to do something doesn't mean that he will want to do it in February. We have seen a child make an error of giving a large dose of insulin that the parent knew nothing about. We have seen children come in for an office visit with a week of blood glucoses running higher than 300 mg/dL, and the parents had no idea that the problem existed. Parents must continue to supervise. Even the most highly motivated children and teenagers who appear to be doing very well make mistakes and misjudgments.

> CASE STUDY. Jocelyn L. is 15 years old and has been handling most of her own diabetes management for several years, gradually taking on increasing responsibility. At her regular office visit she displayed a picture-perfect blood glucose record, with three to four monitoring results listed for every day and all of the counts between 70 and 120. We asked to see her meter, and Jocelyn said that she had forgotten it. "Oh, no," her mother contradicted, "it's in the car, I'll go get it." Jocelyn wished that she wouldn't. The meter showed that no counts had been taken for 6 weeks. "It needs a new battery," Jocelyn offered in weak defense. But we knew that the meter was fine.

We see circumstances like Jocelyn's all too often. Some children will stick to their story despite the contradicting evidence. Most will eventually be truthful, and it is important to give them an opening to do so and reinforcement for telling the truth. In our experience, threats or a punitive attitude are rarely effective. "Everyone gets tired of doing blood sugars, and some people make them up," you may say. And then, "I'm really glad you've been able to be so honest with me." Some parents will collude with their children to cover up problems. We saw one child whose mother insisted that she was giving him all his injections. In private, he confided to us that this was not the case.

Some children hate to monitor; we often see this in teenagers who view monitoring as an extra load of homework, a disagreeable chore. It can be helpful for the parent to step in and serve as stenographer for the child, even though the child is capable of the task. It is also important not to assume that because a child or teen is adherent in one area, he is adherent in all. We see, for example, children who take all their shots and do their fingersticks but don't record the results of the monitoring. We see children who are meticulous with shots and monitoring but don't watch what they eat.

Quick learning is one of the gifts of childhood for some children, and it is not unusual for children, still in a learning mode, to pick up information, techniques, and understanding more easily than their parents. Often we will pitch the education to these children. When parents or children have learning difficulties, there are a number of techniques that can be employed:

> Sometimes just keeping language simple and descriptive can be helpful. Rather than talking about Regular and NPH types of insulin, for example, a clinician might call the two types "clear" and "cloudy."

> For families who have trouble with arithmetic, a tape mark on the syringe to mark the level to be drawn up can be helpful.

> Families who have trouble reading might want to differentiate their day and night doses with a picture of a sun and a picture of stars, respectively.

It is crucial that families understand what they are doing and why they are doing it if they are going to maximize control of diabetes, and clinicians must make every effort to help families achieve this. For example, when discussing how to determine an insulin dose, the clinician should not be satisfied simply with a correct assessment of a dose but should also ask the parent and/or child to go over the decision-making steps that led to the assessment, to ensure that the reasoning and calculations are accurate.

Sometimes clinicians incorrectly assume that families who have lived with diabetes for several years are more knowledgeable about the condition than they actually are. Knowledge gaps occur, even when patients and families have been through education programs, as the following striking example illustrates:

> CASE STUDY.   Barry L. is 14 years old and has had diabetes for 6 years. He and his family have been through two diabetes education programs and thus have been exposed to much information about diabetes. But it is likely that they absorbed this information in an abstract way, without actually applying it to the management of Barry's disease. We realized this during a discussion of meal planning and insulin dosage. "If he eats more food, does that mean he needs more insulin?" Barry's mother asked, indicating to our clinic staff that the family needed another educational initiative that would definitively apply the theories of diabetes management to the specifics of Barry's life.

Home nursing care can be very helpful to families that have difficulty mastering the basics of diabetes management. In some cases, a longer than usual hospitalization in a long-term facility is indicated for educational reasons. While some parents may never be capable of the intensive type of management that other parents practice, many of these parents are highly motivated to help their child and do very well with straightforward management.

6

Insulin

The central cause of insulin-dependent diabetes is insulin deficiency, and all management of the disease is related to compensating for this deficiency. Despite continuing technological advancements, replacement of insulin with currently available methods is not truly physiologic. Unfortunately, we have no perfect method of insulin replacement to offer to our patients.

However, with all its imperfections, modern insulin therapy offers life, health, and even normalcy to most individuals with diabetes. Before the discovery (in 1921–22) that insulin could be used to treat diabetes, the prognosis was grim—and brief—for most people with diabetes. Once the diagnosis was made, the life expectancy of a young person with diabetes was less than a year. Treatments such as bleeding, administration of opium, and even eating large amounts of sugar (to replace what was lost in the urine) were tried, with no success. The one treatment that seemed to extend the lives of people with diabetes was "undernutrition," which—as practiced with some patients—was tantamount to starvation. It was true that maintaining patients on barely subsistence caloric and carbohydrate intakes decreased blood glucose levels, but eventually these patients died too, emaciated and starving.

The discovery of insulin was a dramatic and life-saving breakthrough for people with diabetes, as the following history, described in Michael Bliss's book *The Discovery of Insulin* (Chicago: University of Chicago Press, 1981), illustrates.

CASE STUDY.   Elizabeth Hughes was born in 1908, a child of privilege and social standing. Her father was Charles Evans Hughes, who served at various times as governor of New York State, U.S. Supreme Court justice, and U.S. secretary of state. Elizabeth had a normal and healthy girlhood, but when she was about 11 or 12, she began exhibiting symptoms of polyuria and polydipsia. In the spring of 1919, weak and lethargic, she was diagnosed with diabetes by Frederick Allen. Dr. Allen was a leading proponent of starvation therapy for people with diabetes.

At the time of her diagnosis, Elizabeth was 4 feet 11½ inches tall and weighed 75 pounds. After initial therapy of 1 week of fasting, Dr. Allen put her on a 400- to 600-calorie-per-day diet, with 1 day's fasting each week. After several weeks, he raised her food intake to 834 calories a day. Her weight dropped to 55 pounds, and she was allowed 1,250 calories daily. Elizabeth was eating primarily lean meats, eggs, lettuce, milk, some fruit, and vegetables that had been overboiled (to remove carbohydrates).

Despite her ordeal, Elizabeth was an outgoing, well-spoken, and even cheerful adolescent. She did not know that her diagnosis was a death sentence, her starvation regimen a tortuous extension of the dying. When she was 13, she weighed little over 50 pounds and was a semi-invalid at Dr. Allen's clinic in the Adirondacks.

By the late summer of 1922, Elizabeth was clearly losing her battle. She was 5 feet tall and weighed 45 pounds. But finally Dr. Allen had another treatment to offer her. His colleague in Toronto, Frederick Banting, had documented blood glucose normalization after injecting diabetic dogs (whose pancreases had been removed) with a pancreatic extract he called "insulin." He was beginning experiments on a few patients who had little other hope of survival. Elizabeth traveled with her mother and her nurse to Toronto, where Dr. Banting immediately started her on insulin and increased her diet.

Elizabeth was given 1 cc of insulin twice a day, and the glucose almost immediately cleared from her urine. The girl knew that this new medication had brought her back from the edge. "Oh, it is simply too wonderful for words, this stuff," she gushed to her mother in a letter later that month.

Elizabeth's progress was straightforward, but there were complications. No one knew what dosages of insulin were appropriate, potency varied from batch to batch, and impurities caused painful injections and lumps and numbness. "I feel like a pincushion," she wrote her mother. But she continued to do well. Her hypoglycemic reactions were mild, and she was delighted with the molasses candy that Dr. Banting gave her to treat them.

Elizabeth returned home to Washington after 4 months with Dr. Banting and threw herself into life as a normal girl—a normal girl who gave herself insulin injections every day. She graduated from Barnard College in 1929, married a year later, and went on to have three children. Her husband was a prominent lawyer; she was active in civic affairs and volunteer activities and was a world traveler. In later life, she showed no evidence of complications of diabetes. She died in 1981 of a sudden heart attack, at the age of 73.

THINKING LIKE A PANCREAS

The underlying goal of insulin replacement is to try to match insulin levels to what the pancreas would produce if it were healthy. This depends upon all the factors that have been introduced above—the type and amount of food intake, physical activity, stress, and other physical influences such as illness. Children or teens with diabetes, and their families, must take over the role of the pancreas and learn to think like a pancreas. This requires figuring out which insulins should be used, when, and in what quantities; and how they should be delivered (syringe or pump). Blood glucose levels must be monitored frequently to determine how dosage decisions are working and whether they need to be adjusted.

Insulin can be given only by injection, either intravenously, intramuscularly, or subcutaneously. The subcutaneous route is used for daily management. Insulin cannot be given orally because it is a protein that would be broken down by intestinal enzymes into small peptides with no biologic activity.

All insulin now sold in the United States is designated U-100, meaning that there are 100 units of insulin in each milliliter. Older preparations of

U-40 and U-80 are no longer available. Special insulins for patients who have insulin resistance are available in U-500, but these are rarely needed in the management of diabetes.

This means that all insulin syringes are now manufactured for U-100 insulins. However, syringes come in several different sizes—25 units, 30 units, 50 units, and 100 units—and are available from a number of manufacturers. Needles are becoming increasingly fine (higher-gauge). They also come in two lengths (see fig. 6.1).

Precision and accuracy are very important when injecting insulin, and the syringe must be well made and well marked. The 25-unit syringe (most likely to be used for a small child) has 0.5-unit markings, 30- and 50-unit syringes have 1-unit markings, and 100-unit syringes have 2-unit markings (fig. 6.1). It is important that everyone in the family who has any involvement with insulin injections be familiar with the unit markings on the syringe and know what they mean and how to read them.

CASE STUDY.   Katie R., aged 6 years, was given her insulin injections by her mother. Her mother had been using a 50-unit syringe with every unit marked. She was drawing up 2 units of Regular and 3 units of NPH, measuring by counting lines on the syringe rather than reading the numbered markings. When the pharmacy gave her a 100-unit syringe, which has markings every 2 units, she continued to count lines. This meant that she was giving double doses. This continued for about 1 month, with Katie experiencing mild to moderate episodes of hypoglycemia. The problem was detected during Katie's first appointment with our team, when parents or patients actually demonstrate step by step for our nurse educator exactly how they draw up insulin and give injections.

SOURCES OF INSULIN

In the past 20 years, improvements in manufacturing technology have resulted in increasingly purified insulins. There are currently two companies supplying insulin in the United States: Eli Lilly and Novo Nordisk. Lilly dominates the U.S. market, with Novo Nordisk more prominent in Europe. Their insulins are equivalent, and there is no difference in quality between them. In general, however, it is recommended not to mix brands of insulin.

In the past, most insulins were extracted from the pancreases of animals

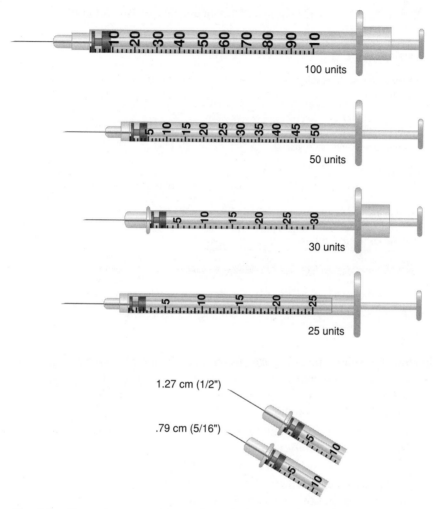

100 units

50 units

30 units

25 units

1.27 cm (1/2")

.79 cm (5/16")

Fig. 6.1. The syringe capacities and needle lengths used for insulin injections (actual size).
Drawn by Jacqueline Schaffer.

(cows and pigs). Human insulin became available in the late 1970s, dovetailing with the tools of modern diabetes management. Today, the vast majority of people in the United States with insulin-dependent diabetes use human insulin. Beef insulin is virtually never used any longer because it is more antigenic than pork or human insulins. Human and pork insulin have very similar chemical structures, with a difference of only one amino acid.

Table 6.1.   **Timing and Duration of Action of Different Types of Insulin**

	Onset	Peak	Duration
Rapid onset			
Lispro	15 min	30–60 min	3–4 hr
Regular (crystalline; soluble)	30–60 min	2–4 hr	4–6 hr
Semilente	1–2 hr	2–5 hr	8–12 hr
Intermediate acting			
NPH (isophane)	2–4 hr	6–10 hr	10–16 hr
Lente (insulin-zinc suspension)	2–4 hr	8–12 hr	12–20 hr
Long-acting			
Ultralente (extended insulin-zinc suspension)	6–10 hr	8–15 hr	18–24 hr
Combinations			
70:30 (70% NPH, 30% regular)	0–1 hr	dual	12–20 hr
50:50 (50% NPH, 50% regular)	0–1 hr	dual	12–20 hr

Source: Modified from American Diabetes Association, *Intensive Diabetes Management* (Alexandria, Va.: ADA, 1995), 53; and P. Chase, *Understanding Insulin-Dependent Diabetes Mellitus,* 8th ed. (Denver, 1995), 49.

Note: Timing and duration are based on doses of 0.1–0.2 units of human insulin per kilogram of body weight, injected in the abdomen.

Human insulin is manufactured using recombinant DNA technology with the human insulin gene, which provides for a virtually unlimited supply of insulin and sidesteps the problems of limited animal supply.

Human insulin may be faster-acting, with an earlier peak and shorter duration than animal insulins. Occasionally, in some people with diabetes, even the longest-duration human insulins will not last through the night, and pork NPH or pork Ultralente are used for improved overnight coverage. (Certain religious dietary laws may preclude the use of pork insulin for some patients, but this is rarely an issue today, with human insulin readily available.)

TIMING AND DURATION OF INSULIN ACTION

The different types of insulin available are listed in table 6.1, beginning with the fastest acting and ranging to the slowest acting.

1. The fastest-acting insulin on the market is lispro, a new insulin marketed by Lilly under the trade name Humalog. It has been on the mar-

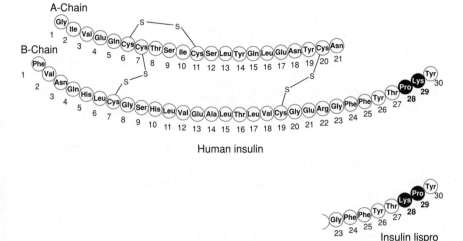

Human insulin

Insulin lispro

Fig. 6.2. *Above:* human insulin molecule; *below:* portion of the lispro molecule that differs from human insulin.
Drawn by Jacqueline Schaffer.

ket since August 1996. Lispro is a modified Regular insulin constructed by reversing two of the amino acids, lysine and proline, in the B-chain of the insulin molecule (fig. 6.2). While the usual Regular molecules aggregate in hexamers, this amino acid reversal decreases the aggregation, so that the molecules aggregate only as dimers. Thus they are easier to dissociate and more rapidly absorbed. Lispro begins working in about 15 minutes, its peak effect occurs in 30 to 60 minutes, and it is largely gone within 3 to 4 hours. It mimics natural human pancreatic insulin secretion much more closely than Regular insulin does.

2. Regular insulin was, until very recently, the fastest-acting insulin available. Regular—which is called "Regular" because it is unmodified pancreatic insulin—begins working about 30 to 60 minutes after injection and has its peak effect 2 to 4 hours after injection; most of it is gone in 4 to 6 hours.

3. Semilente is another short-acting insulin. It is slower than Regular and is uncommonly used in the United States. It begins working within 1 to 2 hours after injection, peaks at 2 to 5 hours, and is gone 8 to 12 hours after injection.

4. NPH (Neutral Protamine Hagedorn) is an intermediate-acting insulin.

("Neutral" refers to the pH, "protamine" is the added protein that slows down the absorption rate, and "Hagedorn" is the name of the scientist who developed it.) Human NPH begins acting 2 to 4 hours after injection and peaks between 6 and 10 hours after injection, and its duration is 10 to 16 hours. Its wide range of action is reflected in its variability of action from person to person.

5. Lente is similar to NPH in onset, but its peak and duration are a little bit later.

6. Ultralente is the longest-acting insulin. It probably begins working between 6 to 10 hours after injection. It does not have a pronounced peak, but its main action is 8 to 15 hours after injection, and it is gone in about 18 to 24 hours.

7. Pre-mixed combinations of types of insulin are also available. These include a 50-50 NPH-Regular mix and a 70-30 NPH-Regular mix.

When and how to use these different insulins, either alone or in combination, will be discussed below.

TYPICAL INSULIN DOSES

Because the timing and duration of action of each insulin can be described only by an approximate range, it is difficult to make assumptions about exactly how an individual patient will react to different types and doses of insulin. Clues about how to adjust the dosage for each individual come from accurate and frequent blood glucose monitoring by the patient. Some guidelines can be suggested, but this is done with the caveat that each regimen must be individualized.

Most children before the onset of puberty need daily insulin doses that total about 0.75 unit to 1.0 unit per kilogram of body weight. Puberty and the adolescent growth spurt tend to increase this requirement by about 25 percent. The average adolescent needs about 1.0 to 1.2 units of insulin per kilogram of body weight per day. The exception to this is during the honeymoon period, because of the endogenous insulin that is present. Dosage requirements during the honeymoon period can drop to less than 0.5 unit per kilogram of body weight per day.

Patients on insulin pumps will often require only about 75 percent of what their daily doses were when they were on injections. This is probably because the pump allows a more physiologically efficient delivery of insulin.

When a child is first diagnosed, we estimate a daily dose that is appropriate for her age and pubertal stage and usually begin on a typical two-shot-a-day regimen. In most cases, this means that two-thirds of the total dose is given in the morning and one-third is given before dinner. Each shot will contain both Regular and NPH, in a proportion usually ranging from approximately one-third Regular and two-thirds NPH, to half Regular and half NPH.

For example, an 11-year-old girl weighing 40 kilograms (88 lb) will be started on 0.75 unit of insulin per kilogram of body weight per day, or a total of 30 units per day. She will be given a dose of 20 units in the morning and 10 units before dinner. The morning dose will consist of about one-third (6 units) of Regular insulin and two-thirds (14 units) of NPH; the evening dose will be about half that amount in the same proportion (3 units of Regular and 7 of NPH).

This is the starting point, and then adjustments will be made depending on what the blood glucose monitoring indicates. Most newly diagnosed children and teens with diabetes will be in the hospital (either as inpatients or in a day hospital program) when their regimen begins, with professional resources readily available for guidance and counsel. If insulin is begun in an outpatient program, close supervision and intensive education are needed. An outpatient program requires a large staff, with personnel available for consultation 24 hours a day. We think that the initial stage of managing the insulin regimen is usually an excessive burden to put on families without giving them the security and resources of the hospital setting for a couple of days. Often parents are frightened by the diagnosis of diabetes, and the protective atmosphere of the hospital helps them to adjust to the life changes this diagnosis means.

Changes to insulin doses are usually made in increments or decrements of 10 percent, in response to blood glucose levels. If a major adjustment is needed—as in the case of a child whose blood glucose rises above 400 mg/dL—a change larger than 10 percent can be made. Doses are also adjusted in relation to the amount of carbohydrates consumed. One unit of insulin usually covers from 10 to 20 grams of carbohydrates, but this is variable. A child who is very sensitive to insulin, or a small child, might need 1 unit or less for every 25 carbohydrate grams, while a person who is relatively insensitive to insulin might need 1 unit for every 5 grams. This concept is discussed more fully in chapter 7. Generally, thin people need less insulin per gram of carbohydrate, as do young prepubertal children. Children who are very physically active also need less.

When blood glucose is out of the target range, one tool, the empirical "1,500 rule" developed by Dr. Paul Davidson, can help to determine the sensitivity factor—how much insulin is needed to get the blood glucose into the target range (P. Davidson, "Bolus and Supplemented Insulin," in *The Insulin Pump Therapy Book*, ed. L. Fredrickson [Los Angeles: MiniMed, 1995], 59–71). The "1,500 rule" is particularly helpful for patients on insulin pumps. According to this formula, divide the number 1,500 by the current total daily insulin dose in units to determine the decrease in blood glucose produced by 1 unit of insulin. For example, the 40-kilogram child described above, who gets 30 units a day, would divide 1,500 by 30 to calculate how many milligrams per deciliter 1 unit of insulin will lower the blood glucose. In this case, 1 unit of insulin will lower the blood glucose about 50 mg/dL (1,500 divided by 30).

These calculations can be very useful in setting up sliding scales of insulin doses which also factor in the amount of carbohydrates being covered. Sliding scales can be used both for pumps and for multiple daily injections, but familiarity with regimens and the cognitive understanding that comes with experience are usually necessary before most families can determine doses with this degree of sophistication.

> CASE STUDY.   Dwayne L. is 13 years old and weighs 45 kilograms (99 lb). His total daily dose of insulin is 30 units. When his monitoring indicates that his predinner blood glucose is 245 mg/dL, about 125 above the top end of the target range, he and his parents use the 1,500 rule to determine how much he needs to increase his insulin dose to lower his blood glucose to a more acceptable level. Dividing 1,500 by 30 (Dwayne's daily dose) tells Dwayne and his parents that 1 unit of additional insulin will lower his blood glucose by 50 mg/dL. Since Dwayne needs to lower his blood glucose by 2.5 times that amount, he adds 2.5 units of Regular insulin to his predinner dose. Continued monitoring will indicate the effects of this change and whether it should be continued, or adjusted further.

It is likely that lispro, the new fast-acting insulin, will substantially change the way in which clinicians and people with diabetes use insulin. Time will tell how this insulin, which is absorbed quickly and also wears off quickly, can best be used. Certainly recommendations about timing of insulin injections before mealtimes are changing with the use of lispro. It is too soon to know what the role of lispro will be—whether it will become the insulin of choice for use in pumps, for example, or for use by people taking multiple daily injections. It may end up having an important but specialized and relatively limited role, or it may end up nearly supplanting the use of Regular insulin.

The bottom line about adjusting insulin doses is that it requires a dual effort:

> ➤ Try to determine at what time(s) of day the blood glucose is out of the target range.
> ➤ Work to adjust the insulin dose that affects that time of day, keeping diet and exercise relatively constant.

TYPICAL REGIMENS

Before modern diabetes management, many people were treated with one shot a day of animal insulins—a combination of NPH and Regular, or Lente and Regular. With the advent of modern diabetes management, including multiple blood glucose checks per day and regular monitoring of glycohemoglobin levels, everyone has become aware of how difficult it is to regulate blood glucose and keep it consistently within target ranges on just one shot a day. (The exception to this is during the honeymoon period, when one shot a day may be sufficient to achieve good control.)

Today the most typical regimen for children and teenagers is a two-shot-a-day regimen, with a combination of NPH and Regular or lispro injected in the morning before breakfast and again in the evening before dinner. The goal of this regimen is for the morning Regular or lispro to primarily cover breakfast and for the morning NPH to cover lunch and a midafternoon snack, with some residual still left to partly cover dinner. The dose of Regular or lispro before dinner covers that meal and part of the before-bedtime snack, and the evening NPH is for the snack and coverage during the night.

There are several advantages of this two-shot-a-day regimen. It is relatively simple to follow, and the injections are scheduled at times of day when children are usually home with their families, thus avoiding the need for injections in the middle of the day when children are at school. Children and teens may do well on a two-shot-a-day regimen.

However, there are some pitfalls. The child or teen is locked into a morning NPH dose, and thus if her lunch is late or she doesn't eat enough lunch, if she gets extra exercise during the day, or if her afternoon snack is small, she is at risk of becoming hypoglycemic. Conversely, if the child is very hungry at lunch and eats more than normal, if she is having an unusually sedentary day, or if she has an unusually large afternoon snack, she is likely to become hyperglycemic in the afternoon. Another disadvantage is that the evening NPH dose may not provide sufficient coverage until morning. Often, evening doses of NPH or Ultralente do not cover the dawn phenomenon (see chapter 8), the early-morning glucose rise.

Supervising this two-shot-a-day insulin regimen with a four-times-a-day monitoring regimen provides the information necessary to fine-tune the process. The goal of the morning Regular or lispro is to cover breakfast and keep the prelunch blood glucoses in the target range; the goal of the morning NPH is to keep predinner blood glucoses in the target range. The goal of the Regular or lispro at dinner is to keep the pre–bedtime snack blood glucose in the target range. The goal of the dinnertime NPH is to keep morning blood glucose in the target range without producing hypoglycemia in the middle of the night. Progress toward these goals can be assessed by monitoring

> ➤ upon awakening;
> ➤ before lunch;
> ➤ before dinner; and
> ➤ at bedtime.

Monitoring is always done before an injection is given, so that the result can help determine the size of the dose. If monitoring often indicates that the evening NPH is wearing off too early during the night, we recommend stepping up the regimen to three doses a day: NPH and Regular or lispro in the morning, Regular or lispro at dinner, and NPH at bedtime. Another alternative is to continue the Regular or lispro at dinner but switch from human to pork NPH, which may have a longer duration. This switch is more likely to be effective with younger children. A third alternative is to substitute Ultralente for the dinner NPH.

Doses of Regular or lispro can be adjusted daily on the basis of blood glucose monitoring results. However, decisions about longer-acting insulins need data from 2 or 3 days of monitoring, so that patterns can be observed before adjustments are made.

CASE STUDY.   Juan S. awakens every morning with his blood glucose above 200 mg/dL. His nighttime blood glucose levels, measured just before his bedtime snack, are in the target range. There are three possible explanations for the problem: (1) The evening insulin is wearing off before morning. This can be particularly noticeable in teens who are sleeping late on non–school days but don't have the problem when they awaken early for school. (2) The evening insulin dose is too low. (3) The evening insulin dose is too high, and the blood glucose has dropped low and rebounded. This is called the Somogyi phenomenon (after the physician who first described it), but recent studies suggest that this rebound occurs rarely and is less likely to be a factor than had been previously thought.

To troubleshoot the problem and differentiate among the several possible causes for the morning hyperglycemia, Juan's family should do an overnight blood glucose panel, taking readings every 2 to 3 hours for two nights. This might mean a very sleepy child, but it is not necessary that these readings be done on two consecutive nights. Usually weekends or non–school nights are best for the overnight panel. This information will indicate which of the following scenarios is associated with the rise in blood glucose:

- ➤ The blood glucose stays between about 100 and 150 mg/dL until about 3 A.M., then gradually rises. This means that the insulin dose is adequate but wears off too quickly, or that the dose is not sufficient to cover the dawn phenomenon. The initial options are to give human NPH at bedtime (and just the Regular or lispro at dinner), to use pork NPH at dinner, or to use Ultralente at dinner.

- ➤ Blood glucose that was in the target range before the bedtime snack rises steadily and is 250 mg/dL or higher for most of the night. The solution to this is to simply raise the dinner NPH dose. It is generally safe to raise doses by about 10 percent at a time. Changing the dose incrementally will usually allow achievement of the target goal without overcorrection. Whenever evening or bedtime insulin doses are adjusted, overnight blood glucose levels should be checked.

- ➤ The blood glucose drops to a low level, below 60 or 50 mg/dL, but then rebounds quickly through the night. This is a less common occurrence. One solution is to lower the evening insulin dose. Again, a 10 percent change is usually safe for the first step. In the pediatric age group this will often mean changes of 0.5 unit or 1 unit, and even smaller changes for very young children. However, if the overnight blood glucose remains low, larger changes will be needed.

MORE COMPLEX REGIMENS

The more complex regimens in use today are primarily regimens that use a basal dose of insulin—usually NPH or Ultralente—to provide a constant low level of insulin, and supplement the basal dose with Regular or lispro to cover meals. In this type of regimen, NPH or Ultralente can be given twice a day (at breakfast and at dinner or bedtime) or once a day at either of these times. Regular is usually given about 30 minutes before a meal and lispro just before the meal. This is similar to the philosophy underlying the use of pumps, which will be discussed in the last section of this chapter.

An example of stepping up the regimen to get better coverage is the case of a teenager who gets out of school at 3 P.M. and comes home, ravenous, to eat a turkey sandwich, three bananas, and a pile of pretzels—a snack that is larger than many people's dinner but is not unusual for a hungry teen. If he raises his morning NPH dose to cover his snack, it might peak too early in the afternoon, resulting in a low. He might also become hypoglycemic if one afternoon he doesn't want to eat as much. The more physiologic approach—doing what the pancreas does—is to cover the snack with another injection of Regular or lispro shortly before the snack. The size of the dose depends on the child's size, what he is going to eat, and what his blood glucose level is.

Another regimen consists of injections of Regular or lispro before breakfast, lunch, afternoon snack, and dinner, plus Ultralente or NPH at dinner or bedtime. Multiple daily injections allow for tighter control. Tighter control, as the results of the Diabetes Control and Complications Trial have shown, means a healthier life with fewer long-term diabetes-related complications.

In summary, patients and families need to consider the following factors in planning and deciding on insulin doses:

> what the blood glucose level is now;
> planned food intake, particularly carbohydrates;
> planned exercise following the meal or snack; and
> how this dose has worked previously in similar circumstances.

VARIABILITIES OF INSULIN ABSORPTION

There are a number of factors that affect the rate of insulin absorption, which in turn contributes to variability of blood glucose levels and potential difficulty in achieving control. These include the site at which the injection is given, how deeply the insulin is injected, the ambient temperature, and physical activity.

Insulin is absorbed most rapidly when it is injected in the stomach, followed in order by the arms, the legs, and the buttocks. The speed of absorption is a function of the amount of fat at the site and the vascularity of the site. If injected deeply into the muscle, the insulin is absorbed more rapidly. This may be hard to avoid in small children without much body fat.

In hot, sunny weather, insulin may be absorbed more rapidly. Exercise and activity also increase the rate of insulin absorption. If a child or teen injects insulin into her leg and then goes out and runs, it may be absorbed more rapidly.

Families can use this information to their advantage. When insulin should be absorbed more slowly—at night, for example—a slow absorption site such as the buttocks can be used. If more rapid absorption is desired—for example, at breakfast—the insulin should be injected into the stomach or the arm.

In the past, it was recommended that injection sites be rotated every day to prevent lipoatrophy and lipohypertrophy. With today's highly purified insulins, skin problems are much less common, and people can use the same area day after day without adverse effects. We often suggest using one area for morning injections and another for evening injections. This does not mean using the same dime-sized site, however. If the arms are the morning site, for example, the area used for injections should be the entire surface of the lateral upper arms.

We encourage parents of children and teens with diabetes to let the child choose the injection site as much as is practical. Children with diabetes often believe that they have little control over this disease and that, in fact, it controls them. Letting them choose the site of injection can be a form of empowerment. Children should not be forced to use a site they don't like and should be permitted to choose a site they prefer as often as possible. That doesn't mean that they should use the same exact site over and over again until it gets lumpy, but we recommend letting them choose, for example, an arm rather than a leg, if that is their preference.

Leakage is another factor that can affect insulin levels and thus blood glucose levels. It is not uncommon for insulin to leak out of the needle track when the needle is withdrawn. If monitoring reveals unexpectedly high or variable blood glucose, with no apparent explanation, it may be that some of the insulin is escaping through leakage. If there is wetness on the skin after the injection, insulin is leaking. Significant amounts of insulin can be lost this way.

To avoid leakage, the person giving the injection should let go of the skin pinch before or after pushing in the plunger on the syringe, and then wait 5 to 10 seconds before removing the syringe after the injection. Leakage may also be reduced by pushing the syringe plunger in very slowly.

ASSISTIVE DEVICES

There are devices on the market that make insulin injections easier for some patients:

Cartridge devices, such as the NovoPens manufactured by Novo-Nordisk and the B-D Pen made by Becton Dickinson, work very well for people on multiple daily injections. These are very popular in Europe. The insulin is packed in prefilled cartridges. Some teenagers, needing an extra dose to cover added snacks when they go out for the evening, prefer to use cartridges rather than vials of insulin and syringes. A cartridge device, which allows a person to dial in the dose and then inject, may be more acceptable than a syringe in a school setting, where syringes may be associated with illicit drug use. Cartridges are available with different insulin types and with a Regular-NPH mix.

Air injectors are needleless injectors that inject the insulin under very high air pressure. These may serve a purpose for some children with a severe needle phobia, but we do not generally recommend these devices for a number of reasons. For one thing, they are expensive, and some insurers do not cover them. In addition, some patients say that they hurt as much as a needle, and they can cause bruising. Fractions of units cannot be drawn up. Also, absorption may not be predictable, since some of the insulin may go into muscle and some may spray onto the skin. However, some patients have had good results with these devices, and newer models are improved.

The case of Ryan D. taught us a little about the leakage and misinterpretation that might occur.

CASE STUDY.   Ryan D., aged 8 years, used an air injector. He weighed 22 kilograms (48.5 lb), and his daily dose was 16 units of insulin—10 units in the morning, and 6 at dinner. His father injected him. Giving Ryan his evening dose (3 units of Regular, 3 of NPH), Mr. D. saw a great deal of insulin left on the skin and falsely assumed that little or none had penetrated the skin. He then administered another dose at a higher pressure. Ryan had a hypoglycemic seizure in the middle of the night.

INSULIN INFUSION PUMPS

The first reports on the use of pumps for continuous subcutaneous insulin infusion (CSII) were published in the late 1970s. Studies showed that it was possible to achieve excellent blood glucose control with blood glucose levels consistently in the target range by combining use of the pump with conscientious home blood glucose monitoring. Pumps were initially used by adults and then by teenagers, and now we are using pumps with some children as young as 9 years of age. For many patients, pump therapy has the potential to allow much smoother diabetes management than does any other regimen.

Currently, two companies—MiniMed and Disetronic—manufacture pumps, and both have toll-free telephone lines to answer questions about these sophisticated devices. The pumps have slightly different features, but they function in exactly the same way. The choice depends upon individual preference, and we do not recommend one over the other.

When an insulin pump is used, a small needle attached to a long catheter is inserted into the skin and secured in place with tape for 2 or 3 days at a time. The insertion sites are usually on the abdomen or thigh. The pump is about the size of a deck of cards and holds the insulin supply, usually about 3 days' worth. The pump is usually placed in a pocket or clipped to the patient's waistband, like a beeper. Less commonly, a patient may strap the pump to his calf with an elastic strap. (Some implantable pumps are also available, but these remain investigational and are used with adults.) The pump, which is connected to the needle by the catheter, pumps insulin steadily. Pumps are now technologically sophisticated, with fail-safe features that eliminate the problem of overinfusion of insulin.

To date, insulin pumps do not have a "brain." All of the brain work must come from the user. The pump is not an artificial pancreas. It is an open-loop system that does *not* get feedback about blood glucose levels and make necessary adjustments. The person with diabetes must do the monitoring and apply the information acquired from monitoring to dosage decisions to achieve optimal use of the pump.

There is no minimum age for successful use of the pump. Maturity is more important than the actual age of the child. This is a very individual issue, and the decision to use or not to use a pump will be based on the child's and family's ability to deal with all the complexities of pump management. Candidates for use of the pump must be highly motivated. They must have a family group available to help with pump management, as well as experienced and available professional backup. They must be comfortable with wearing the pump, which may be visible, although small. They must have excellent problem-solving abilities and be willing to monitor blood glucose a minimum of four times a day and communicate the results to a management team. They also must be able to manage (either through insurance coverage or personal resources) the financial outlay for a pump, which will cost at least $4,000.

The major reasons that people choose pumps are to achieve better control and to have more flexibility in their schedules. DCCT results showed that patients with pumps achieved equal—but not better—outcomes compared to those who followed multiple daily injection regimens, and many patients changed from multiple daily injections to pumps and vice versa. Pump users must be aware, however, that using a pump is actually more difficult than a typical regimen and requires more work than a two-shot-a-day regimen. It requires more cognitive decisions about altering the insulin dose on the basis of food intake and physical activity, and more monitoring. Some children and teens, despite being told many times that life with a pump will *not* be easier, don't believe this and think that a pump will help them forget that they have diabetes. But this is not the case. People who want a pump because they think it will make them forget about having diabetes, or because they think that it will require less work in management of diabetes, are unlikely to use a pump successfully and will be very disappointed with pump use.

The first requirement of candidates for pump use is that they be very highly motivated about diabetes management in general. They must understand all the issues about diabetes management and must be able to monitor, record, and communicate to their parents and clinicians. They must understand that life with the pump will not be easier and will, in fact, require more work as a trade-off for the better control and increased flexibility the pump will allow. We require that our pump candidates use a demonstrator pump with saline solution for 3 to 7 days (along with their usual injections) to see how they like it. Before getting a pump, they will also meet with a representative from the pump manufacturer, who may well use an insulin pump himself.

A basic principle of insulin administration via a pump is the distinction between the basal infusion rate and bolus doses. This distinction can be illustrated by an injection regimen that uses NPH or Ultralente to provide basal coverage and pre-meal injections of Regular or lispro as the bolus to cover food intake. The difference is the continual infusion of basal insulin through the pump, using Regular or lispro insulin only. The basal rate can be adjusted depending on individual needs, in order to keep the person's blood glucose level steady when she is not eating. This infusion rate is preprogrammed by the user, and multiple basal rates can be used. For example, more insulin may be needed in the early morning hours to cover the dawn phenomenon (see chapter 8).

Because of the continual infusion provided by a pump, only Regular or lispro insulin is used in pumps. The standard recommendation with Regular insulin has been to adjust basal rates about 2 to 3 hours prior to blood glucose changes. As use of the shorter-acting lispro becomes more prevalent, these patterns may be revised.

The multiple basal rate function in pumps makes the pump an ideal method of covering the dawn phenomenon. For example, an individual may program the pump to infuse the basal insulin at the rate of

> ➢ 1 unit per hour from 8 A.M. to 8 P.M.;
> ➢ 0.6 units per hour from 8 P.M. to 4 A.M.; and
> ➢ 0.9 units per hour from 4 A.M. to 8 A.M.

The infusion of additional insulin in the early morning hours averts the hyperglycemic dawn phenomenon. This effect can be dramatic to observe through close monitoring: some children's blood glucose levels will remain constant through the night but begin a steady rise in the morning, even before they have eaten breakfast. The rise is believed to be related to overnight hormonal activity. For further discussion of the dawn phenomenon, see chapter 8.

Bolus doses are given to cover meals and snacks. The size of each dose is determined by the blood glucose level, the carbohydrate content of what will be eaten, the time of day, and the amount of physical activity that may be undertaken.

When therapy with an insulin pump is started, the total daily dose is calculated by first reducing the current daily dose by about 25 percent. Then this amount is divided in half, with half for the basal rate and the remaining half for boluses. We begin by using a constant basal rate over 24 hours, and modify this on the basis of blood glucose levels, especially overnight. The total bolus dose should then be divided by the number of meals and snacks and appropriately apportioned. It is usually simpler to initiate pump therapy by figuring three meals a day of equal carbohydrate content and equal bolus doses at each meal. Adjustments are then made on the basis of blood glucose levels and amount of food intake.

It is not always easy to predict which patients will do well with pumps, which patients will have more difficulty with them, and what external factors will come into play, as the following case studies illustrate.

> CASE STUDY.   Tyler S. was diagnosed with diabetes when he was 6 years old, and as he approached age 10, his diabetes control became increasingly difficult. His blood glucose levels were often over 200 mg/dL, his glycohemoglobins averaged about 10 percent (normal: 4.5 to 6.1%), and he was on relatively high insulin doses. He was on a multiple-shot regimen to try to achieve better control, and when he was 13 we started thinking about a pump. He wanted to try it.
>
> Tyler began on the pump when he was 13½; at that time, his height was 159 centimeters (62.5 in.), his weight was 49.7 kilograms (110 lb), and he was in midpuberty. His daily insulin dose was about 60 units. Before he started to use the pump, he was on four shots a day and his control still was suboptimal. He started on pump therapy, with a 3-day hospitalization to learn how to use the pump. His blood glucose levels improved markedly, and on lower doses of insulin.
>
> Four weeks after starting with the pump, Tyler removed the insulin syringe reservoir from the pump mechanism and injected himself with 100 units of Regular insulin. This occurred after an argument with his parents about a subject unrelated to diabetes management. We met the family in the emergency department. Tyler was treated with intravenous glucose quickly enough to avert a serious hypoglycemic reaction, but the impulsive action clearly showed an underlying psychopathology and we referred Tyler for counseling. The psychological evaluation did not indicate that he

was suicidal, but we took him off the pump, taking a position of caution, not punishment or lack of trust. Nine months later, he, his therapist, and his parents all felt that his behavior remained too impulsive to begin pump therapy again, although his glycemic control remained suboptimal.

CASE STUDY.   Whitney C. had a more positive outcome with a pump. Diagnosed when she was 15 years old, she was 155 centimeters (61 in.) tall and weighed 49 kilograms (108 lb), with adult sexual maturation. Whitney and her parents quickly mastered the technical and cognitive aspects of diabetes management. Whitney is a competent and composed young woman. She monitored her blood glucose levels regularly and adjusted her insulin doses, factoring in carbohydrate intake and blood glucose levels. She also had autoimmune thyroiditis and hypothyroidism, and maintained normal thyroid levels on l-thyroxine. She maintained excellent glycemic control, with glycohemoglobin levels between 5.9 and 7.1 percent (normal: 4.5 to 6.1%).

Whitney started on the pump when she was 16, and her subsequent glycohemoglobin levels were 6.0 and 5.2 percent. She maintained basal rates of about 0.5 units per hour, with boluses of about 1 unit of insulin for every 20 carbohydrate grams. She is able to follow up on her decisions and refine her decision-making according to the results of her monitoring. She pays close attention to diabetes management but does not make it the major focus of her life. She does well in school, participates in sports, is active in other school activities, and has a boyfriend. Her weight has remained stable on the pump. Her control has been excellent on the pump, except for two or three episodes of deteriorating control, which never lasted more than a day and were associated with fights with her boyfriend.

CASE STUDY.   Sammy S. is a younger child who has done well with a pump but also illustrates some of the problems with pump management seen in younger patients. Diagnosed with diabetes when he was 5 years old, he had 4 years of good control, with glycohemoglobin levels in the 6.5 to 7.0 percent range. He started on a pump at his own request just before his 10th birthday, hoping for more flexibility in management.

Sammy is a bright and motivated boy, but he sometimes forgets to take his bolus dose before lunch and comes home from school with very high blood glucose, above 500 mg/dL. This is a continuing intermittent problem of which Sammy is aware. As he grows older, this has been occurring less and less frequently.

7

Dietary Management

with Madeline Michael, M.P.H., R.D., C.D.E.

Dietary management of children and teens with diabetes is complex and intensive—and critically important. The underlying principle of diabetes management is balancing insulin doses with insulin requirements, and these requirements are primarily determined by the amount and type of food a person eats. Food plays a major role in determining blood glucose levels, a fact that became apparent with the earliest understandings of diabetes.

It was once taught that the basic dietary principle of diabetes management was to avoid sugar. But advanced understandings of food metabolism have shown that all carbohydrates—not just sugar—have similar effects on blood glucose. This has led to a basic change in philosophy and practice regarding sugar, which unfortunately has led to substantial confusion, not only on the part of families living with diabetes but also on the part of health professionals. With the time-honored tradition of "no concentrated sweets" removed from the dietary rule book, the question of what to teach people with diabetes and their families about food and diabetes has become more complicated. The days of handing out lists of forbidden foods and preprinted diet patterns are gone—but what can clinicians offer to replace them?

Chapter 3, "Survival Skills for Patients and Parents," presented a brief discussion of philosophies of eating and meal planning. This chapter presents the details of how to apply these philosophies to daily life. Clinicians will have varying degrees of involvement in dietary management, depending on their interest, training, and available time. It is our experience that only the physician or nurse with extensive nutritional training, background, and interest is qualified to handle the details of day-to-day meal planning, particularly in the case of active growing children, whose nutritional requirements are constantly changing.

Few busy clinicians have time for this. It is a job for a professional, and we recommend ongoing consultation with a dietitian for the dietary management of children and teens with diabetes. The dietitian is an important part of the diabetes management team. Continuing consultation with a dietitian for meal planning is important, especially in the initial period after diagnosis, and at least annually thereafter so that meal plans can be redesigned to suit changing needs.

Nonetheless, every clinician involved with treating the child or teen with diabetes needs a basic understanding not only of the underlying nutritional principles but also of some of the finer points of applying those principles to daily living. As has been emphasized throughout this book, each individual and family with diabetes must determine the type of regimen with which they feel most comfortable and must continue to adapt and fine-tune it to fit a changing lifestyle. Hopefully, being flexible and teaching people to use insulin to cover what they are eating will help to avoid the food problems and potential eating disorders that are sometimes seen in individuals who spend too much time thinking about food and feel that they are denying themselves what they want to eat.

The most important principle of dietary management for people with diabetes is that they should be attentive to all food and beverages that are consumed and cover them with insulin. Conversely, all insulin doses must be balanced by food, and once a child or teen has had an insulin dose, he will risk a potentially dangerous low if he skips a meal or snack. Food intake is part of the formula that is a vital component of effective diabetes management.

Nutritional recommendations for people with diabetes have evolved gradually over time. The model food plan for a child or teenager with Type

1 diabetes is basically the same healthy diet that any child or teen should eat, with adequate calories and nutrition for normal growth. This means that it is low in fat—particularly saturated fat—and high in fiber, with plenty of fresh fruits and vegetables.

Food strategies for people with diabetes have run the gamut. In the past, the "diabetic diet" was based on commonly held beliefs that seemed to make sense, although they lacked scientific research to back them up. Today's recommendations are based more solidly on clinical experiences and published research.

Before the discovery of insulin in 1921, starvation diets were prescribed in an effort to prolong life. After insulin treatment was initiated, a high-fat, low-carbohydrate approach was used. Since that time, the recommended percentage of calories from fat has declined from 70 percent to current recommendations of less than 10 percent of calories from saturated fat. As the recommendations for fat have decreased, the recommendations regarding the percentage of calories from carbohydrate have increased.

In previous years, restrictions on "simple" carbohydrates were based on the belief that in the person with diabetes, sugars were absorbed too rapidly, resulting in hyperglycemia. The consumption of "complex" carbohydrates was encouraged, as it was believed that they were digested and absorbed more slowly, resulting in a much slower blood glucose rise. The rule of "no concentrated sweets" for anyone with diabetes was easy to teach and understand. Health professionals simply gave people with diabetes lists of food to avoid. However, complying with this diet was not always easy. And people with diabetes often assumed that if a food did not contain sucrose, they could eat it in unlimited quantities.

Questions such as "How much sugar is too much?" or "What is the effect of more complex carbohydrates?" led to research that essentially dispelled the myth that a food plan with no concentrated sweets led to better blood glucose control. Modern diabetes management recognizes that sucrose can be a part of a meal plan for children and teens with diabetes, within the context of a healthy diet.

In 1994, the American Diabetes Association revised its nutritional recommendations for people with diabetes. The new guidelines promote a better understanding of the role of diet in diabetes management and emphasize that an individualized approach, taking lifestyle and blood glucose goals into account, is important for success.

The ADA's five goals of medical nutrition therapy for diabetes parallel the goals that have been presented in other contexts throughout this book:

1. Maintain blood glucose levels as close to normal as possible by balancing food intake with insulin.
2. Aim for optimal serum lipid levels.
3. Give infants, children, and adolescents adequate calories for maintaining normal growth and development. A meal plan or "diet" should not be calorie-restricted, unless obesity is a problem. Regular monitoring of a child's growth curve provides valuable information about adequacy of the diet.
4. Prevent and treat the acute complications of Type 1 diabetes, including hypoglycemia, short-term illnesses, exercise-related problems, and long-term complications.
5. Improve overall health through optimal nutrition. The diet for a child with diabetes is designed as a healthy diet that the whole family can enjoy and benefit from.

MEAL-PLANNING APPROACHES

A meal plan should be based on the child or adolescent's usual food intake and should be used as a basis for integrating insulin therapy into the usual eating and exercise pattern. The timing of meals is as important as their content. Eating at consistent times synchronized with the peak action of insulin is essential for good blood glucose control. For most children, this means eating three meals and three snacks spaced throughout the day. Older children may be able to skip the midmorning snack. Once children are on a consistent eating pattern, efforts should be made to adjust their insulin to their usual eating habits, rather than restricting food for a hungry child or, conversely, forcing food on a satiated child, in order to improve blood glucose control.

There are many possible approaches to achieve a consistent eating plan. No single plan is right for everyone. A plan should be based on the level of education, motivation, and lifestyle of the child and her family. While we try to emphasize flexibility, the philosophy of a food "prescription"—eat the same amount at the same time every day—makes it easier for some patients to maintain control, particularly in the early period after diagnosis when they are learning to cope with their condition. Exchange lists (explained later in this chapter) provide a convenient guide for substitutions, so that someone with diabetes does not have to eat the same thing every day, even when on a relatively fixed meal plan.

Clinicians can usually get a sense of what a family can or cannot man-age. If we have the sense that all the calculations and figuring are too much for a family to deal with—particularly at the time of diagnosis—we put the patient on a two-shot-a-day regimen with a set eating routine and a set in-sulin dose. We ask them to try to keep physical activity constant, and de-sign as simple a regimen as possible and let them begin on that. Then, as they gain knowledge, experience, and confidence, they become able to master a more flexible regimen. The speed at which this transition can be accomplished varies greatly from family to family.

From the most rigid regimen, with the same amount of food at the same time each day and the same amount of insulin at the same time each day, the next step might be to always eat the same amount but adjust the insulin in relation to exercise and blood glucose readings. A somewhat more flexi-ble intermediate regimen would have the child eating relatively constant breakfasts and lunches but more variable dinners. At the far end of flexibil-ity is the schedule of the child or teen who uses an insulin pump, and whose regimen does not prescribe a set amount of food. The child could fast all day and be covered by the basal infusion, or she could eat every hour, covering the food intake with boluses.

Beth's eating plan is an example of a plan with intermediate flexibility.

> CASE STUDY.   Beth C. is 12 years old and has had diabetes for 4 years. She weighs approximately 45 kilograms (100 lb), and her daily insulin dose is approximately 38 units, 25 in the morning and 13 at night. She consumes about 2,200 calories a day, of which 50 percent are carbohydrates, amounting to 275 grams. Her carbohydrates are roughly divided so that she eats 70 grams at each meal (breakfast, lunch, and dinner) and 30 grams at each of two snacks. She know that she needs a unit of fast-acting insulin for every 15 grams of carbohydrates.
>
> Beth takes NPH and lispro at breakfast, adjusting the dose of the short-acting insulin in relation to the carbohydrate content of the meal. For breakfast, she usually has a large bowl of cereal, juice, and a slice of toast, equaling 70 to 75 grams of carbohydrate. She covers this with about 5 units of lispro. On a morning when she decides to have bacon and eggs and one slice of toast, a meal containing only 15 grams of carbohydrate, she takes only 1 unit of lispro. However, she has less flexibility with lunch, which will be covered by the morning NPH dose. At dinner she will have another dose of lispro, adjusted according to the amount of carbohydrates in her meal. If she eats a large bowl of pasta with green peas, a meal loaded with

carbohydrates, she will need a higher dose of lispro than she would need to cover a steak and salad. (Carbohydrate counting is explained in detail below.)

Special circumstances require a flexible approach, as Lisa and her family learned at her first Thanksgiving after being diagnosed.

CASE STUDY. Lisa P., who is 8 years old, has very good control on two insulin shots a day. She takes a combination of Regular and NPH before breakfast and then again before dinner, which is usually at 6:30 P.M. Her family was not sure how to handle her insulin needs on Thanksgiving Day, when dinner would be at 3 P.M., the usual time of Lisa's after-school snack. We suggested that the most flexible solution was to give Lisa the morning dose as usual; give a dose of Regular or lispro before Thanksgiving dinner, to cover the carbohydrates in the dinner; and then give the evening NPH at the usual time. Since dinner would be so early, Lisa and her parents would need to make sure that she ate her usual bedtime snack to avoid an overnight low.

Lisa didn't know exactly how much food she was going to eat at Thanksgiving dinner, but she and her family were able to make a reasonable estimate. If she used lispro, it would be possible to cover the carbohydrates *after* they were consumed, but it would still be important to keep track of exactly what Lisa ate.

A basic approach in providing nutrition education is to introduce patients and/or their families to the U.S. Department of Agriculture's Food Guide Pyramid. The Food Guide Pyramid (fig. 7.1) organizes foods into groups, with the broad base of the pyramid (grains, beans, and starchy vegetables) representing the largest number of servings per day. The other groups on the pyramid, from bottom to top, are fruits and vegetables; then milk and meat; and finally fats, sweets, and alcohol. The higher up the pyramid a group is, the fewer servings per day there should be from that group. The Food Guide Pyramid can provide basic information needed for families of very young children with diabetes, newly diagnosed families, or families without the technical mathematical skills needed for more complex meal-planning approaches.

The labeling that the Food and Drug Administration currently requires on most foods provides a useful tool for determining the meal plans for a child or teen with diabetes. Families need to learn how to read food labels,

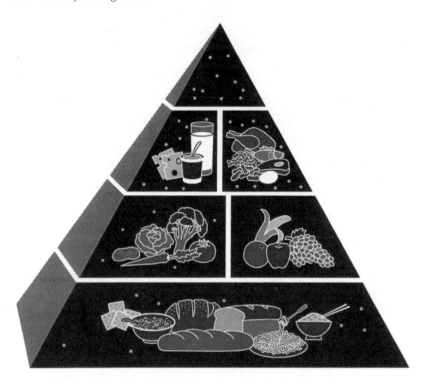

Fig. 7.1.   The Food Guide Pyramid, a guide to daily food choices.
The Food Guide Pyramid, *Home and Garden Booklet 252 (Washington, D.C.: U.S. Depart-ment of Agriculture, Center for Nutrition Policy and Promotion, 1996), 3. Available online at http://www.usda.gov/fcs/library/961001.pdf.*

Table 7.1.   **Sample Portion Sizes for Infants, Children, and Teenagers**

Food Group	Infant	Toddler and Preschooler	School Age	Teen
Milk	16–24 oz	2–3 cups	2–3 cups	4 cups
Breads and cereal	4 servings, ¼ of adult serving each, or 1–2 tbs	4 servings, ¼ of adult serving each, or 1 tbs per year	4 exchange-size servings	4 exchange-size servings
Fruits and vegetables	4–5 servings, ¼ of adult serving or 1–2 tbs	4–5 servings, ¼ of adult serving or 1–2 tbs	4–5 exchange-size servings	4–5 exchange-size servings
Meat and protein	2 servings, ½ oz each	2–3 oz	2–3 oz	4–5 oz

Source: Adapted from Betty Pace Brackenridge and Richard Rubin, *Sweet Kids: How to Balance Diabetes Control and Good Nutrition with Family Peace* (Alexandria, Va.: ADA, 1996).

Table 7.2.   **Basic Guidelines for Diet in Children with Type 1 Diabetes**

Eat meals and snacks at regular times.
Eat about the same amount of food every day.
Try new foods.
Don't skip meals.
High-protein foods may help to provide a slow rise in blood glucose and should
   be included as part of a bedtime snack to help prevent overnight hypoglycemia.

Source: Adapted from *The First Step in Diabetes Meal Planning* (Alexandria, Va.: American Diabetes
Association and American Dietetic Association, n.d.).

how to evaluate what a serving size is, and how to determine the amounts of carbohydrate in each serving.

Despite the FDA requirements, it is still necessary to be wary of food labeling and to examine how each particular food item can fit into the food plan of a child or teen with diabetes. Some foods are labeled "dietetic" or "diabetic," but that does not necessarily mean that they are appropriate for someone with diabetes. Such labeling may refer to the form of sweetening—corn syrup or sorbitol rather than sucrose, for example. Also, "fat-free" does not mean calorie-free, and "natural" does not mean sugar-free.

Sample portion sizes for children are shown in table 7.1. A brochure, *The First Step in Diabetes Meal Planning*, published by the American Diabetes Association and the American Dietetic Association, provides not only information about the pyramid and serving sizes but also basic diabetes meal-planning guidelines, emphasizing that a healthy diet is the first step in taking care of diabetes. Table 7.2 lists some of the guidelines recommended in this brochure for children with diabetes.

EXCHANGE LISTS

The Exchange Lists for Meal Planning, commonly referred to simply as *exchange lists*, provide a more in-depth approach to meal planning and are one of the most widely used systems in diabetes dietary education (see table 7.3). The basic principle of exchange lists is that foods within a single category can be substituted for each other in comparable quantities.

The exchange lists group foods into categories based on the amounts of carbohydrate, protein, fat, and calories they contain. This system, used in combination with an individualized meal plan, provides a guide for the amount and types of food to be included in meals and snacks. The ex-

Table 7.3.   **Nutritional Values of Food Exchanges**

Food Group	Nutritional Value per Exchange			
	Carbohydrate (g)	Protein (g)	Fat (g)	Calories
Carbohydrates				
Starch	15	3	1 or less	80
Fruit	15	—	—	60
Milk				
skim	12	8	0–1	90
low-fat	12	8	5	120
whole	12	8	8	150
Other carbohydrates	15	varies	varies	varies
Vegetables	5	2	—	25
Meat and meat substitutes				
very lean	—	7	0–1	35
lean	—	7	3	55
medium-fat	—	7	5	75
high-fat	—	7	8	100
Fats	—	—	5	45

Source: *The Exchange Lists for Meal Planning* (Alexandria, Va.: American Diabetes Association and American Dietetic Association, 1995).

change lists were revised in 1995 to reflect the changing recommendations regarding sugar and changes in the products available in the marketplace.

The new exchange lists now contain three general groups of foods: carbohydrates, meats and meat substitutes (protein), and fats. The carbohydrate group contains five categories: starches, fruits, milk, vegetables, and "other carbohydrates." The starch group includes bread, cereals, grains, pasta, and starchy vegetables such as corn and potatoes. The fruit group includes fruit and fruit juices. The vegetable group includes nonstarchy vegetables such as carrots, broccoli, and zucchini. The "other carbohydrates" category contains foods that were traditionally restricted, such as desserts and high-sugar foods including syrups and jelly. The addition of the "other carbohydrate" category helps to dispel the notion of "bad" foods and communicates the most current recommendations—that sugar and sweet foods can be incorporated into a healthy diet.

Foods in the starch, fruit, milk, and "other carbohydrate" categories contain approximately 12 to 15 grams of carbohydrate per serving and can be interchanged for one another. Vegetables contain approximately 5 grams of carbohydrate per serving and are not usually counted as carbohydrates unless three or more servings are eaten at one time. The meat group is divided into four categories: very lean, lean, medium, and high fat. Many young children dislike meat and prefer cheese or peanut butter, which are included in the high-fat meat category. The fat group is divided into three categories—monounsaturated, polyunsaturated, and saturated—and includes the obvious sources of fat such as butter and margarine, in addition to less well recognized sources of fat such as salad dressings, bacon, and sour cream. Portion sizes are listed for each food included in a category. Exchange lists also provide information on "free foods" (foods with less than 5 g of carbohydrate or less than 20 calories), combination foods, fast foods, and the reading of labels.

These exchanges can help provide the flexibility that children with diabetes and their families need to integrate a balanced diet into a busy lifestyle. The goal of the exchange lists is twofold: to keep carbohydrate, fat, and protein intake consistent at a particular meal or snack; and to allow for choice and variety when planning what to eat. A consistent dietary intake will help lead to a more consistent blood glucose pattern, which will allow for meaningful insulin adjustments.

> CASE STUDY. Kristie H. is 16 years old and has had diabetes for 5 years. She has an active social life and over the past few years has assumed increasing responsibility for managing her own diabetes. After school she often goes with her friends to the shopping mall, where she faces many possible food choices. In addition, her parents work late many evenings, and she is responsible for preparing her own meals. She would like to cook but is afraid that this would interfere with her afternoon activities and completing her homework in the evenings. She wants to learn how to incorporate some of her favorite mall foods and some frozen convenience foods into her exchange diet. In addition, she is often too rushed on school mornings to eat a bowl of cereal and wants to find breakfast foods that she can eat quickly. Table 7.4 shows an exchange pattern for a 2,200-calorie diet and a sample meal plan that was based on Kristie's usual diet. This plan, developed in conjunction with a dietitian, allowed Kristie to continue to participate in the social activities that were important to her and have a balanced diet.

CARBOHYDRATE COUNTING

With many of our children and teens, we find that carbohydrate counting is another meal-planning approach that allows increased flexibility. The rationale for carbohydrate counting is based on three assumptions:

Table 7.4. **Sample Meal Plan for a 2,200-Calorie Diet**

Meal Plan for: Kristie   Date: _____

Dietitian: _____   Phone: _____

			Grams	Percent
		Carbohydrate	300	55
		Protein	80	15
		Fat	73	30
		Calories	2200	

Time	Number of Exchanges/Choices	Menu Ideas	Exchanges

7:30 A.M.	5 Carbohydrate group
	  3 Starch
	  1 Fruit
	  1 Milk
	0 Meat group
	1 Fat group
		8 oz low-fat fruit yogurt
		4 oz orange juice
		1 low-fat granola bar
			= 3 carbs
			= 1 fruit
			= 1 carb

11:30 A.M.	4 Carbohydrate group
	  3 Starch
	  1 Fruit
	      Milk
	  ✓ Vegetables
	3 Meat group
	1 Fat group
		Sandwich
		  2 slices bread
		  3 oz turkey
		  lettuce, tomato, mustard
		³⁄₄ oz pretzels
		1 orange
			= 2 carbs
			
			= 1 carb
			= 1 fruit

3:00 P.M.	5 Carbohydrate group 1 Fat	1 cup frozen yogurt or 1 large soft pretzel Diet drink	= 3 carbs

6:00 P.M.	5 Carbohydrate group
	  3 Starch
	  1 Fruit
	  1 Milk
	  ✓ Vegetables
	3 Meat group
	2 Fat group
		Lowfat french bread pizza
		Salad, 1 tbsp fat-free dressing, free
		½ cup carrots
		17 grapes
		8 oz skim milk
			= 3 carbs, 3 meat, 2 fat
			
			= 1 fruit
			= 1 carb

9:00 P.M.	3 Carbohydrate group	½ cup low-fat pudding 8 oz skim milk	= 2 carbs = 1 carb

1. Carbohydrate is the major determinant of postprandial blood glucose.
2. Approximately 90 percent of carbohydrate appears in the blood as glucose within a couple of hours after eating.
3. Smaller amounts of protein are converted to glucose at a much slower rate. Only foods containing carbohydrate are counted.

The child's system of carbohydrate counting can vary from simple to complex, depending on the needs and lifestyle of the individual. Carbohydrate counting has been classified into three levels: basic, intermediate, and advanced. The American Diabetes Association and the American Dietetic Association have jointly published three education booklets outlining each level of carbohydrate counting.

Our families consult with a dietitian to determine goals for carbohydrate choices or grams of carbohydrate at each meal and snack; these goals are based both on the child's usual diet and on a plan for a healthy eating pattern. For the most basic level of carbohydrate counting, a consistent amount of carbohydrate is consumed at each meal and snack daily. The exchange lists are a good reference for learning how to count carbohydrates. However, in carbohydrate counting—unlike the exchange system—foods from the meat (protein) and fat groups are not counted because they contain little or no carbohydrate.

This does not mean that fat and protein cannot influence blood glucose. A high-fat meal may slow stomach-emptying time and result in a delayed rise in blood glucose. Protein may also influence blood glucose, but not until many hours after a meal. These nutrients also contain calories (9 calories per gram of fat, and 4 calories per gram of protein and carbohydrate) that will influence weight gain.

A single portion from the carbohydrate group contains about 15 grams of carbohydrate. Weighing, measuring, and reading food labels are necessary skills that will help children and families accurately determine the amount of carbohydrate in foods. Keeping food records and testing blood glucose regularly are important steps for moving up to the intermediate level of carbohydrate counting.

In the intermediate level of carbohydrate counting, people with diabetes learn to identify patterns in their blood glucose levels which are related to the foods that they eat, their insulin dose, and their activity level. Target goals for blood glucose levels should be set. Grams of carbohydrate, blood glucose readings, and physical activity need to be recorded daily to detect patterns that will allow for adjustment of insulin and progression to the most advanced level of carbohydrate counting.

The third level in carbohydrate counting, the use of an insulin-to-carbohydrate ratio (or the reverse, a carbohydrate-to-insulin ratio), allows the most flexibility in the timing and size of meals and snacks. The amount of insulin is adjusted on the basis of the number of grams of carbohydrate eaten. This level of carbohydrate counting is designed for individuals practicing intensive diabetes management by taking multiple daily injections or using an insulin pump.

Fairly good blood glucose control is necessary to advance to insulin-to-carbohydrate ratios. Before advancing to this level, an approximate basal dose of insulin (either Regular or lispro infused through a pump, or an injected intermediate- or long-acting insulin) and a sliding scale of Regular or lispro should be determined. Basal (or background) insulin is the insulin that is required to keep blood glucose under good control when fasting; it is the amount of insulin needed to balance hepatic production of glucose to maintain glucose homeostasis. Bolus doses should provide enough short-acting insulin to bring blood glucose levels back to the target range within a maximum of 3 to 4 hours after a meal.

The insulin-to-carbohydrate ratio is largely determined on the basis of trial and error and good recordkeeping. To accurately determine the ratio, at least 2 weeks of food, activity, and blood glucose records should be reviewed. The amount of carbohydrate eaten during a meal is divided by the number of grams of carbohydrate covered by 1 unit of insulin. For example, for a person needing 1 unit of insulin for every 15 grams of carbohydrate, a meal containing 75 grams of carbohydrate would require 5 units of insulin (75 divided by 15).

If blood glucose levels are above the target range following a meal, a different ratio is needed; thus, a larger dose of insulin is given to get the blood glucose back to the target range. A low insulin sensitivity means that more insulin is needed to cover a meal; conversely, a high insulin sensitivity means that less insulin is needed.

This ratio can vary tremendously from one person to another, depending on an individual's insulin sensitivity. A person with high insulin requirements will need 1 unit of insulin for every 5 grams of carbohydrate eaten. Conversely, a person who is very insulin-sensitive may need only 1 unit of insulin for every 25 grams of carbohydrate. The amount of insulin that a person needs can vary during the course of a day. One unit of insulin may cover fewer grams of carbohydrate at breakfast than at other meals because of a variety of factors including the dawn phenomenon, lower activity levels, and lack of recent previous boluses while sleeping.

Carbohydrate counting offers people with diabetes the potential for improved blood glucose control and a more flexible lifestyle. It requires skill and practice to perfect, but most people who use insulin-to-carbohydrate ratios think that the payoff in achieving better blood glucose control is worth the time and effort invested. Carbohydrate counting will usually require multiple sessions with a dietitian and significant time and effort at home, keeping and reviewing records and adjusting insulin until a correct ratio is determined. Anyone practicing carbohydrate counting should be comfortable with her mathematical skills and have a high level of motivation to keep track of all the different variables.

> CASE STUDY.   Donald R. is 17 years old and has had diabetes since he was 6. He enjoys playing competitive sports and usually plays soccer after school. He does not want to eat a large snack before practices and games, because he believes that this slows down his performance. However, he finds it difficult to prevent low blood glucose levels without eating. Another problem develops when, after exercise, he is extremely hungry and finds it difficult to control his food intake, which results in high blood glucose levels later in the evening.
>
> Donald takes three insulin shots per day but is not satisfied with his blood glucose control. He would like to try an insulin pump so that the varying rates of basal insulin delivered throughout the day would allow him to decrease his basal rate during periods of exercise. He would also be able to vary his caloric intake and the timing of meals, snacks, and insulin boluses to better fit with his schedule and appetite. In preparation for the pump, Donald has kept 2 weeks of food, blood glucose, and activity records and has had three sessions on carbohydrate counting with the dietitian. He has determined that he will require 1 unit of insulin for 8 grams of carbohydrate in the morning and for 12 grams of carbohydrate at other times during the day. A sample record is shown in table 7.5.

Families are usually ready to make the shift from fixed meals and fixed insulin doses to the flexibility of figuring insulin-to-carbohydrate ratios when the following can be demonstrated:

➤ relatively well controlled blood glucose levels;
➤ basal insulin rates that are relatively steady and well adjusted;
➤ a good understanding of how to adjust insulin on the basis of blood glucose levels;

Table 7.5.   Sample Diabetes Self-Care Daily Record

Day of week __Monday__   Date _____

Time	Medication Type	Medication Amount	BG Results	Food Intake Amount	Food Intake Type of Food/Drink	Carbohydrate Information Grams	Physical Activity Type	Physical Activity Amount
A.M. 6:00	R	12	135	2 cups 8 oz	Raisin bran Skim milk	83 12 95	sedentary	
9:00	R	1	156	1	Banana	15		
11:00	R	9	123	1 8 oz 2 1	"Sub" sandwich Skim milk Sandwich cookie Large orange	45 12 20 30 107		
P.M. 3:00	R	2	95	8 oz	Orange juice	30	strenuous	60 min
6:00	R	6	128	2 slices ½ cup 8 oz	Thick-crust pizza Salad Skim milk	60 — 12 72	sedentary	
9:00	R NPH	4 8	142	1 cup 8 oz	Raisin bran Milk	40 12 52		
					Daily Totals	370		

Comments

> ➤ a good understanding of how the different types of insulin act; and
> ➤ understanding of how to adjust insulin or use food to cover exercise (it is helpful to keep exercise constant as one begins to understand how much insulin is needed to cover how much carbohydrate).

The change to the use of insulin-to-carbohydrate ratios can be made gradually and situationally, or not at all. A fair amount of experimenting may be necessary, which means frequent blood glucose monitoring to ascertain the results of the experimentation. There is a spectrum of options for family and patient involvement, food choices, and insulin doses and regimens. As families gain more experience, the sophistication and flexibility of their regimen can usually be increased. However, this is not always a straight path. You may find that a sophisticated multishot regimen supervised by the parents works very well for a child when he is 9 and 10, but that when the child reaches adolescence and wants more independence and management on his own, he is not ready for the flexibility that his parents have been managing.

Finding the best path requires knowing your patient and maintaining comfortable communication with him and his family. The child must be able to say, "It's too much—I can't do this now"; and the clinician should be able to help him figure out the problems and work through them. Sometimes people will say, "I've mastered this, and I'm ready to move on to something more complicated." More frequently, though, you are likely to hear, "You're asking me to do too much."

THE GLYCEMIC INDEX

While we do not often use this method of meal planning with our patients, it is helpful for clinicians to know a little about it. The glycemic index (GI) is a ranking of foods based on comparison of the postprandial blood glucose response to each food to the blood glucose response to a reference food, which is often bread or glucose.

A low-GI diet has been proposed as another method that could be used in the dietary management of diabetes. However, past criticisms of the GI have noted that although it may be useful when comparing single foods, the addition of other foods, as in a meal, makes the usefulness of the rating uncertain. Potatoes may have a high glycemic index, for example, but most people do not eat only potatoes for a meal. They also eat meat, vegetables, and dairy products.

Recent studies have demonstrated some predictability in the glycemic index when foods with different GIs have been incorporated into a mixed meal; however, this remains controversial. Given the complexity and un-proved long-term benefits of the GI method, questions remain about implementing a low-GI diet. Books and tables on the glycemic index have been published and can serve as a resource for patients interested in incorporating low-GI foods into their meal plan.

WEIGHT CONTROL AND INTENSIVE THERAPY

People who are about to embark on a more intensive insulin schedule are usually aware of the benefits that better blood glucose control can bring. The Diabetes Control and Complications Trial proved that better control leads to fewer long-term complications. However, it is not so well known that tighter blood glucose control also may result in the potential for weight gain and increased episodes of hypoglycemia.

This weight gain can be due to a number of factors. Poor blood glucose control results in the loss of sugar in the urine. Once control is improved, these calories are no longer "lost" and become available to be stored, thus causing weight gain. Also, individuals practicing intensive therapy with a pump or multiple daily injections may think that carbohydrate counting is "eating whatever you want." It may be easy to forget that protein and fat contribute calories even if you are not "counting" them.

In the past, people with diabetes sometimes experienced poor blood glucose control after overeating, which resulted in a negative feedback toward overindulging and self-imposed restrictions on food intake. Once a person becomes adept at balancing insulin and carbohydrates, overeating may not result in high blood glucose levels; this elimination of a negative reinforcer may give the green light to further splurging.

Finally, as blood glucose levels approach normal physiologic levels, the chances of hypoglycemia increase. An increased number of hypoglycemic episodes will cause a person to eat more food to counteract the lows. Decreasing the number of hypoglycemic episodes is important to prevent weight gain and to promote better blood glucose control.

TREATING HYPOGLYCEMIA

We recommend treating hypoglycemia with "neutral" foods that are not tempting to children, such as glucose gel or tablets or fruit juice. This will avoid situations in which children become tempted to fake lows or induce them—by extra exercise or skipping a meal, or even by taking extra insulin—in order to be given candy or other sweets.

In the past, there was no other room in the diet for such splurges, and a hypoglycemic episode gave children the opportunity to eat these foods without the usual guilt associated with eating sweets. However, the many parents who gave their children sweets to treat low blood glucose levels often found themselves in the uncomfortable position of being manipulated by the child. Many children become very adept at faking the symptoms of a low. This is most likely to happen when a child feels deprived about not getting what she wants to eat.

Treating hypoglycemia with candy or similar sweets only rewards poor blood glucose control. Also, because a majority of chocolate calories come from fat and protein, chocolate bars may take hours to be digested and absorbed, which results in a slower blood glucose rise at first—when it is needed—but a high blood glucose level hours later. Carrying candy around in case of an emergency is not recommended because the candy often is eaten long before a hypoglycemic event and then is not available when it is most needed.

Using neutral foods to treat a low and including sweeter foods as part of the usual diet rewards good blood glucose control and ensures that a source of carbohydrate will be available when most needed.

Treating hypoglycemia is discussed in detail in chapter 10.

AGE-RELATED FOOD ISSUES

Infants

Infants and very young children with diabetes should be fed on demand. Infants and young children often have erratic eating behaviors that can lead to frequent hypoglycemic episodes if blood glucose goals are set too tightly. Children with unpredictable appetites and eating patterns may need to receive insulin after a meal, instead of before one, with the dose based on the actual amount of food eaten. Now that lispro is available, this is a workable approach.

Infants and young children with diabetes should be fed in the same manner as children without diabetes—on demand or every 2 to 3 hours, depending on the age of the child. They should not be on a fat-restricted diet. No special formula is required, and the only recommended restriction is to limit juice (or sweetened beverages) to 2 to 3 four-ounce servings throughout the day, depending on the age of the child. When problems develop, they are often due to a deviation from normal patterns, as in the case of Colin.

> CASE STUDY.   Colin B. was diagnosed with Type 1 diabetes when he was 9 months old. Because of his young age, Colin's parents were advised not to restrict his diet and to continue to give him his infant formula as well as appropriate foods for his age. It was recommended that they limit juice to no more than 4 ounces twice a day.
>
> Colin and his parents returned to the clinic for a follow-up appointment a month later. They reported that Colin was constantly hungry. A review of his growth chart revealed no weight gain since diagnosis. In further discussion, the dietitian learned that Colin's parents, concerned about high postprandial blood glucose levels, had decided to dilute the baby's formula with water, to produce better blood glucose readings. This resulted in a hungry child who was unable to gain weight because of inadequate caloric intake. The goals for blood glucose were reviewed with the family, and the need for continued growth with an unrestricted diet was emphasized.

Toddlers and Preschoolers

Three meals and three snacks are the mainstay of diet planning for 2 to 6 year olds. The age at which to introduce a systematic meal-planning approach such as exchange lists or carbohydrate counting is variable. Initiating such a plan depends less on a child's age and more on the child's eating habits and cognitive ability.

During the preschool years, children are only starting to develop more predictable eating habits and food preferences, and adhering to an exchange-type diet is challenging. Often parents find that setting a carbohydrate goal for meals and snacks is a realistic option when trying to initiate a consistent diet. Uneaten carbohydrate can be substituted from one group to another, allowing flexibility in the diet while encouraging consistency. In addition to carbohydrate, a protein source should be served at meals and at bedtime to try to prevent overnight hypoglycemia. It is normal for children of this age to go on food "jags," eating the same foods day after day. This type of consistency can often work to a parent's advantage, making it easier to predict insulin requirements.

School-Age Children

Sending a child with diabetes to school can be an anxiety-provoking experience for parents. Children who were at home or in a small group setting, under the watchful eye of a parent or day care provider, are now part of a larger group. The fact that they will be engaging in unpredictable physical activity and eating in an environment that does not allow the previous close attention often leads to well-founded concerns about hypoglycemia. Blood glucose goals should be reevaluated and set at realistic levels, and insulin doses should be adjusted as needed to decrease the likelihood of low blood glucose levels. When planning meals and snacks, and the insulin schedule, parents will have to factor in the child's usual eating pattern, school lunch menus, and the timing and amount of activity at recess, gym, and afterschool sports.

Because of the energy needed for growth, food plans for the majority of children with diabetes should not be restricted in calories. The child's growth should be monitored regularly, using the National Center for Health Statistics Growth Curves, to assess for adequacy of the diet. The Recommended Dietary Allowance gives an approximate estimate of calorie needs for children based on age and weight (see table 7.6). However, a meal plan should also be based on an estimate of actual caloric intake derived from a review of the child's usual diet. Children who are obese may need moderate restrictions in calories to allow for a slower rate of weight gain; for these children, physical activity should be emphasized.

Adolescents

During their teenage years, adolescents take more responsibility for their diabetes care. As they strive for independence and increase their social activities away from home, their meals and snacks are no longer closely monitored by their parents. Risk-taking behavior and concerns about self-image may influence their diabetes self-management.

Many adolescents discover that poor blood glucose control can produce an "easy" weight loss. Particularly for teenage girls, the temptation to eat

Table 7.6.   **Recommended Dietary Allowance for Calories and Protein, Based on Age and Weight**

Age	Calories (g/kg of weight)	Protein (g/kg of weight)
Infants		
0–6 months	108	2.2
6–12 months	98	1.6
Children		
1–3 years	102	1.2
4–6 years	90	1.2
7–10 years	70	1.0
Males		
11–14 years	55	1.0
15–18 years	45	0.9
Females		
11–14 years	47	1.0
15–18 years	40	0.8

what they want and not gain weight may overshadow any concerns about the long-term consequences of poor control and the inconvenience of more frequent bathroom visits.

It is important that adolescents understand that better blood glucose control reduces the risk of long-term complications. However, it is also important to present the negative side. To avoid unpleasant surprises, the issues of weight gain and the possibility of increased episodes of hypoglycemia should be addressed before initiating intensive insulin therapy.

The continued monitoring of growth and glycohemoglobin levels remains important as children go through their teenage years. Questions about "easy" or rapid weight loss, about preoccupation with weight or food, and about food fads or fad diets should be included in history taking. A discussion of the effects of alcohol and its risk of hypoglycemia is also important at this age. Promoting flexibility in choices is important to allow for increased control of food. Carbohydrate counting, along with intensive therapy, is preferred by many adolescents, as it allows for more control not only of the amount of food that may be eaten but also of the timing of meals and snacks.

TROUBLESHOOTING

If a child or teenager is not following the meal plan, it is important to determine the reasons why. The child must have input into designing the meal plan. There is no reason for anyone to feel that a favorite food—chocolate, ice cream, or any other treat—cannot be part of his meal plan. Anything can be included, in moderation.

Children and adolescents should not have to feel hungry when following their meal plans. If a child feels that the amounts of food allotted in her food plan are too small, then the food plan is wrong and must be readjusted so that the child isn't hungry much of the time.

It is part of the clinician's job to lighten the burden that diabetes places on children and teens and on their families. This can take time—more time than many clinicians may usually devote to routine office visits. It means really listening to what patients are saying, and picking up on the undertones. Remember Ellen L., the 10 year old in chapter 3 who threw her syringes and told us that the hardest thing for her about life with diabetes was not being able to eat Oreo cookies. By incorporating Oreos into her meal plan, we lightened her load by letting her know that we understood the daily stresses and challenges of living with diabetes. We could even make her laugh, as we determined the portion. "Do you want a whole bucketful of Oreos?" we joked. But we never would have known that a problem existed if we had not listened, asked, and probed.

Good clinical skills are similar to good parenting skills. You need to listen, to establish self-esteem and trust. Mutual trust is an important part of the clinician-patient relationship.

Clinicians, and families with diabetes, are aiming for the best possible blood glucose control in the context of the total life of each individual. Needs in life will change from time to time, and flexibility is crucial. We must adjust the regimen to meet the child's needs. An example is seen with many of our teenagers, who come home from school at 3 in the afternoon, feeling ravenous, with dinner not scheduled until 6 P.M.. At 3 P.M. they eat a large snack, and their blood glucose subsequently rises substantially if this has not been covered with insulin. If we raise the morning NPH insulin, blood glucose may be low by midafternoon. If we raise the prelunch insulin dose, the teen may be even hungrier after school, and his blood glucose may be lower at dinner. We calculate how much insulin to give and when it should be given in order for blood glucose to be within the target range at dinnertime. Further specifics regarding how this fine-tuning is done are given in chapter 8.

Language and attitudes are very important. We want our patients to come away from their clinic visits feeling good about themselves. A critical, judgmental, tearing-down approach is rarely effective in the long or short run. It never helps to make a person feel negative about herself. Conversely, a caring attitude and empathic language turn this into a win/win situation and can really help young people feel better about themselves. If they like themselves, they will do better not only with diabetes management but with life in general.

However, parents sometimes expect us to be sterner and ask us to "lay down the law," to take the role of disciplinarian. Often this does need to be done, but with a positive tone.

The complexity and difficulty of dietary management for the child or teen with diabetes should not be underestimated. However, it is also important not to lose sight of the fact that adjustments can be made, variables juggled, to accommodate the many facets of the life of an active child or teenager.

> CASE STUDY.   Michael M., 12 years of age, was diagnosed with diabetes about 3 years ago. Generally his control has been good, although his blood glucose levels are sometimes out of the target range, with glycohemoglobin levels that vary between 6.0 and 7.5 percent (normal: 4.5 to 6.1%). He is very active physically, participating in a variety of sports: soccer, baseball, and basketball. In addition to his seasonal afterschool sports activities, he has a period of physical education every day during school, but not at the same time every day. Three days a week, Michael's gym class is the period immediately preceding lunch. This puts him at risk of a low right before lunch.
>
> To compound this problem, on some school mornings Michael just doesn't feel like eating breakfast. This has become a point of contention between Michael and his parents. We advised several possible solutions to resolve the conflict. Michael has been on a three-shot-a-day regimen, taking NPH and Regular before breakfast, Regular at dinner, and NPH at bedtime. On a morning when Michael does not want breakfast, the morning Regular can be reduced. If this coincides with a day when he has physical education class before lunch, the morning Regular can be eliminated altogether. If lunch is late, the morning NPH will also have to be decreased.

8

Fine-Tuning and Sick Day Management

L iving with diabetes is a constant process of fine-tuning the regimen. "She's running high in the morning, what should we do?" a mother will call and ask; or "She's running low at night, what now?" We give our families options and choices and discuss the outcomes they can expect from each course of action. As with almost everything else involved in daily diabetes management, decisions are made in close collaboration between the clinician and the family.

Diabetes management may seem relentless. It means making the necessary adjustments day by day, meal by meal, sometimes hour by hour, with the dual goals of maintaining a normal, active life and consistently keeping blood glucose levels within the target range. This chapter provides some very specific principles, techniques, and examples that demonstrate how to troubleshoot, balance, and fine-tune by adjusting food, insulin, and physical activity to improve blood glucose control in a variety of circumstances.

The adjustments, recommendations, and suggestions that we discuss below can be determined by a number of different people—the primary care physician, the nurse educator, a specialist, or a knowledgeable family member with an excellent understanding of diabetes management. Some primary care clinicians may feel comfortable with the tinkering that fine-tuning involves; others may prefer to enlist the help of a specialist. Our nurse educator is particularly effective in this role. Some parents do it all the time, but others will never be able to do it. Who does what depends upon the skills, knowledge, and experience of each individual.

FINE-TUNING

The two basic principles behind fine-tuning are technical and cognitive. First, accurate recordkeeping is essential—carefully recorded and precise blood glucose results, logged in a way that clearly illustrates emerging patterns and links them to food intake, insulin dose, and physical activity. Second, one must think about what factors could be influencing the blood glucose levels at the times of day or night that are of concern, and figure out what to do about them.

These influencing factors include

> amount, type, and timing of meals and snacks;
> amount, type, and timing of insulin doses;
> amount, type, and timing of physical activity (immediate as well as within the past 10 to 18 hours);
> unusual or unexpected stress;
> illness;
> the injection site; and
> accuracy of dose measurement.

When considering the injection site, it is necessary to consider the exact spot on the body where the shot was given, the possibility of exercise immediately after an injection and the way in which that might have affected absorption, the depth to which the needle penetrated, and the possibility of leakage. To determine problems with dose measurement, consider questions such as: Is it possible that there was an error in measurement? Is it possible that the morning dose was given at night or vice versa? Is it possible that the same dose was given twice, once by one parent and once by the other? Could a dose or part of a dose have been forgotten? Is it possible that the NPH and Regular measurements were reversed?

Sometimes the solutions to problems are complex, but sometimes they can be simple.

CASE STUDY.   Jim P. is a 4 year old who was diagnosed with diabetes 2 years ago. He weighs 16 kilograms (36 lb) and is given insulin doses of 5 units of NPH and 3 to 5 units of Regular in the morning, and 2 units of NPH and 1 to 3 units of Regular in the evening.

One evening Jim's mother called at about 7 p.m., very upset. She had just realized that for Jim's 6 p.m. predinner dose, she had mistakenly given him the morning dose, injecting him with 5 units of NPH and 4 units of Regular, which was more than twice his usual evening dose. What should she do? she asked.

This is the time for Jim to indulge in his favorite dessert, we told her. Then, she should take special care to monitor him before bedtime and should make sure that he got his bedtime snack to prevent an overnight low. In addition, she should monitor him every 2 to 3 hours overnight, until the NPH cleared, which would be near morning.

CASE STUDY.   Danny B. is 10 years old and in a transitional period developmentally, beginning to take responsibility for injecting himself. One evening he gave himself his predinner shot of insulin but somehow forgot to tell his mother this, and she gave him the shot again. It was only after she gave him the shot that Danny said, "Oh, Mom, I already did that."

Again, this was an occasion for indulgence in a favorite dessert. It was a hot summer night, and Danny and his mother wanted to go out for ice cream. We advised her that this would be fine, and that a big bedtime snack and extra blood glucose monitoring were also needed.

Everyone forgets a shot now and then. People are usually mortified when this has happened and embarrassed that they could forget something this important. Keeping record sheets easily accessible—for instance, on the refrigerator or a bulletin board in the kitchen—and making a notation of each shot can help to prevent this forgetfulness. When forgetting becomes repetitive, it is not forgetting, and there are psychological causes that need to be investigated. The clinician can talk, listen, and refer patients or families for further psychological help when necessary.

Administration of incorrect doses and insulin leakage do occur. This may be because of negligence, carelessness, or improper technique. When blood glucose levels are out of the target range and you are looking for the reasons, be sure to consider these possibilities. In our clinic, we have patients or their parents demonstrate to us regularly (once or twice a year, or more often if needed or if the patient is newly diagnosed) exactly how they draw up and inject insulin. Errors of which they are unaware can be detected in this way.

TROUBLESHOOTING THROUGH THE DAY

Various strategies can be employed when trying to diagnose and treat problems that occur throughout the day (see table 8.1).

Morning Lows

If fasting blood glucose is consistently below the target range (70 mg/dL) upon awakening, a change definitely must be made. For a small child, morning levels below this are dangerous and require immediate attention. For an older child, a pattern of lows—for example, lows that occur 3 or 4 days in a row—must be addressed. If there is a low 1 day out of 7, then you can focus on the night before a specific episode and can usually find a specific cause (e.g., a missed bedtime snack) that can be avoided in the future.

A few specific steps are recommended:

First, lower the evening dose of intermediate- or long-acting insulin, NPH or Ultralente. We recommend a decrease of 10 to 20 percent, or sometimes more, depending on how low the morning counts were.

The second step—which can be done simultaneously with the first—is to gather as much information as possible. We instruct families to do overnight blood glucose panels on two nights, checking every 2 to 3 hours during the night. This can be hard on the child and the family, especially if the monitoring is done two nights in a row, but it does not usually need to be done on consecutive nights.

Third, increase the calories in the bedtime snack. Be certain that the snack is nutritionally complex, consisting of carbohydrate, fat, and protein, and not just carbohydrates. Just apple juice (for example) is not sufficient. Pure carbohydrates raise the blood glucose, but they clear quickly. The more complex snack will have more impact on blood glucose levels longer into the night.

Fourth, consider whether there was unusual physical activity during the evening or afternoon before the morning low. We encourage physical ac-

Table 8.1.   **Troubleshooting Lows and Highs**

Lows	Highs
Morning	
1. More information; overnight BG panels 2. Lower evening N or U 3. Increase or adjust bedtime snack	1. More information; overnight BG panels 2. Adjust evening N or U 3. Decrease bedtime snack
Lunch	
1. Lower A.M. R 2. Change A.M. R to lispro 3. Increase breakfast calories and carbohydrates 4. Add or increase midmorning snack	1. Increase A.M. R or lispro 2. Decrease breakfast calories and carbohydrates 3. Decrease or eliminate midmorning snack
Dinner	
1. Decrease A.M. N or U 2. Decrease lunchtime R 3. Change lunchtime R to lispro 4. Increase lunchtime calories and carbohydrates 5. Add or increase midafternoon snack	1. Check midafternoon (presnack) BG: — if low, increase lunch calories and carbohydrates or decrease A.M. N or U, or lunch R or lispro — if high, increase A.M. N or U; add R or lispro at lunch 2. Cover snack with R or lispro
Bedtime	
1. Decrease predinner R 2. Change predinner R to lispro 3. Increase calories and carbohydrates at dinner 4. Decrease evening exercise	1. Increase predinner R or lispro 2. Decrease calories and carbohydrates at dinner 3. Increase evening exercise
Overnight	
1. Decrease P.M. N or U 2. Change P.M. R to lispro 3. Increase bedtime snack and use complex snack	1. Increase P.M. N or U 2. Decrease bedtime-snack calories and carbohydrates

Abbreviations: BG = blood glucose; N = NPH insulin; R = Regular insulin; U = Ultralente insulin.

tivity and don't advise against it at any time of the day. But it is necessary to adjust insulin or food intake to compensate for exercise.

Morning Highs

If the fasting blood glucose is high, a couple of overnight blood glucose panels will help to determine whether the level is high because there was an insufficient evening insulin dose, because the dose is wearing off too early, or because there is a rebound from an earlier low blood glucose.

If the insulin dose is insufficient, the blood glucoses will be high throughout the whole night. The remedy for this is to increase the evening dose of either NPH or Ultralente by about 10 percent. Continue to monitor, and increase the dose another 10 percent if blood glucose levels still remain above the target range.

If the insulin is wearing off too early, blood glucose levels will remain satisfactory until about 3 or 4 A.M. and then will begin to rise. This can also be due to the dawn phenomenon (see below). The options for treating this are to

> ➤ move the predinner dose of NPH or Ultralente to bedtime;
> ➤ substitute pork NPH for the evening dose of human NPH, since pork may be longer-acting;
> ➤ change the predinner dose of NPH to Ultralente.

If the morning low is due to a rebound, the overnight panel will show a low blood glucose level in the middle of the night, with an increase toward morning. As data have demonstrated, however, this is less common than previously thought. The solution to rebounding blood glucose is to decrease the evening NPH or Ultralente in gradual steps of about 10 percent each time, monitoring each change to see what the results are.

Morning Variability

A third possibility in the morning—and the most difficult to figure out and treat—is variable fasting blood glucose levels. If readings are frequently above and frequently below the target range, it is necessary to work on consistency in the amount, type, and timing of the bedtime snack and consistency in the amount, type, and timing of physical activity, particularly in the late afternoon and evening.

It is also important to check for consistency in measuring the insulin dose and in the choice of injection site. In practical terms, this means using the same site for the evening injection every day, and in the case of a small child, it means having the same caretaker draw up and inject the evening insulin dose every day.

Sometimes it is impossible for physical activity to be consistent every day. Consider the example of a 15-year-old girl who plays basketball in league competition three evenings a week. Although she is active on the other days, her activity during the rest of the week is nowhere near the level it reaches on the days of competitive basketball games. The first step is to ascertain whether there is blood glucose inconsistency on active versus less active days, and if so, the next step is to adjust food and insulin accordingly.

For children and teens who are on an insulin pump and experiencing inconsistent morning blood glucose levels, an overnight panel with blood glucose counts every 2 or 3 hours will show at what time during the night the pattern becomes irregular. Since only Regular or lispro insulin is used with a pump, this variability can be treated by addressing the problem 2 to 3 hours before it occurs if Regular is used, or at the time it occurs if lispro is used. For instance, if blood glucose is elevated at 4 A.M., raise the basal rate of Regular starting between 1 and 2 A.M. (or of lispro starting between 3 and 4 A.M.), starting with an increase of 0.1 unit per hour. If that first-step change is not adequate, then continue to re-evaluate on the basis of overnight blood glucose monitoring.

Prelunch Lows

If the blood glucose before lunch is low, lower the breakfast Regular or lispro, usually by 10 to 20 percent; increase the calories or carbohydrates in breakfast; or add or increase a midmorning snack. Regular insulin, even though it is considered short-acting, does have a long decay tail (residual effect). If this is causing the low, a switch from Regular to lispro, in equivalent doses, may be helpful. Because Regular insulin does not start working immediately and peaks a couple of hours after the dose is given, sometimes the morning dose of Regular is sufficient to prevent the postbreakfast high but is too high to prevent prelunch lows.

Sometimes children and teenagers have low blood glucose levels before lunch because of a morning physical education class. This may not be scheduled every day, and activity may be more vigorous on some days than on others, making the exercise difficult to plan for. It is usually effective to add or increase the midmorning snack on the days that gym class is scheduled, or lower the breakfast Regular or lispro dose.

Prelunch Highs

When prelunch highs occur, several options can be tried, alone or in combination. Either raise the morning dose of Regular or lispro, decrease breakfast calories and carbohydrates, or decrease or eliminate a midmorning snack. Which approach to use depends in part on the child's caloric needs. For the heavier child, lower the calories. For the thinner child, increase the insulin.

Prelunch Variability

Again, when variability is the problem, it is important to work on achieving consistency of all of the factors involved: the amount, type, and timing of food, physical activity, and insulin. It is critical to understand the different carbohydrate contents of different foods, even foods with similar caloric contents. A breakfast of ham and eggs may have the same amount of calories as a breakfast of cereal and toast, but the cereal and toast will provide more carbohydrates, thus requiring a higher dose of insulin for coverage.

Applying and adjusting the insulin-to-carbohydrate ratio will address the variations. If you are using 1 unit of insulin per 10 grams of carbohydrates, and the blood glucose level is high, try 1 unit of insulin per 8 grams of carbohydrates. If the blood glucose level is low, try 1 unit of insulin per 12 to 15 grams of carbohydrates.

Afternoon and Dinnertime Variability

The predinner period is the time when even patients who are in consistently good control will most often record highs and lows on their charts. There is often a long stretch of time between lunch and dinner. Much can happen in those hours. When children and teenagers get out of school in the midafternoon, they often are physically active and eat snacks. There are many variables at work, and information about all of them must feed into decisions about insulin doses.

Again, complete and accurate information is the key to troubleshooting. It is important to know what the time span was between lunch and dinner, what the activity level was, and what was eaten for lunch and the afternoon snack.

When predinner blood glucose levels are low, consider lowering the morning NPH or Ultralente, again starting with 10 percent decrements. If the child or teen is taking Regular at lunch, lower the lunchtime dose. Other alternatives are to increase the lunch calories and carbohydrates, or to add a midafternoon snack or increase the size of an existing one. Still another possibility is switching the lunch Regular to the shorter-acting lispro.

To solve the problem of predinner highs, start by getting a midafternoon blood glucose level. If the child or teen is eating a midafternoon snack, measure his blood glucose level before the snack. This is typically the time of day when morning NPH or lunchtime Regular is at its peak, so blood glucose levels may be low at this time. In response to this low, a child may then eat a calorie- and/or carbohydrate-packed afternoon snack, which will raise the predinner blood glucose level above the target. It is easy to make the mistake of raising the morning NPH to prevent this predinner high, thinking that more insulin is needed to cover the afternoon.

Sometimes an extra dose is the answer to predinner highs.

> CASE STUDY. Matthew C., aged 15 years, could not get control of his predinner blood glucose levels, which his monitoring showed were consistently elevated. When we questioned him, we found that after school, at about 3 P.M., he would eat a big snack—for example, a large turkey sandwich, an apple, and a bag of tortilla chips. His morning doses were not sufficient to cover this, leading to the predinner highs. Matthew solved his problem by adding an additional injection of lispro before his afternoon snack, with the dose adjusted according to the amount of carbohydrates in his snack. This brought his predinner blood glucose levels back into the target range.

Some children and teens might not have low blood glucose levels in the midafternoon but still might want a big snack after school. To avoid the predinner high, this snack can be covered by an additional shot of Regular or lispro in the afternoon. This option gives flexibility to the child who does not definitely want to commit in the morning to having a big snack in the afternoon.

If the blood glucose level is high before the midafternoon snack, the options are to increase the morning NPH or Ultralente, or to increase or add lunchtime Regular. Another alternative is to lower the lunch and snack calories and carbohydrates, but that is usually not the best choice for a growing child or teenager.

Bedtime

If bedtime blood glucose (measured prior to the bedtime snack) is low, either lower the predinner Regular, consider a switch from Regular to shorter-acting lispro, increase the calories and/or carbohydrates eaten at dinner, or consider reducing physical activity (although this last choice is usually not recommended).

If bedtime blood glucose is high, increase the dose of Regular or lispro at dinner, lower the calories and/or carbohydrates at dinner, or increase physical activity.

If bedtime blood glucose levels are variable, this should be investigated as for variability at other times of the day: carefully analyze all the factors that could contribute, and monitor blood glucose levels frequently to determine when problems begin to occur.

Overnight

Many parents' worst fear is that in the quiet of the night, while their child sleeps and they sleep, an unobserved low will persist, dropping to dangerous levels that can lead to seizures, coma, brain damage, or even death. It is true that overnight is one of most dangerous times to have low blood glucose, but it is also true that these severe reactions with severe sequelae are rare.

Overnight lows are usually preventable by careful, systematic, and frequent monitoring. Every family should do an overnight blood glucose periodically—maybe once a week, or at least every couple of weeks. Any change in routine should be a trigger for more vigilant monitoring. A parent who thinks that a child, particularly a young child, didn't eat enough at dinner should consider doing a finger-stick between 2 and 3 A.M. If there is any suspicion of an error in dosage, overnight blood glucose levels should be checked.

Overnight lows may be treated by one or more of the following changes: lowering the nighttime dose of NPH or Ultralente; replacing the dinner Regular with lispro, which wears off more quickly; increasing the calories in the bedtime snack and using a more complex snack that contains some fat and protein as well as carbohydrate; or decreasing evening physical activity, which again would be the last choice.

The Dawn Phenomenon

The dawn phenomenon, or early morning glucose rise, is a complex management issue that often requires close monitoring by the clinician and frequent contact with the family. It occurs because of an increase in insulin requirements due to insulin resistance in the few hours before awakening (between approximately 4 A.M. and 8 or 9 A.M.). The early morning hours (11 P.M. or midnight to 3 or 4 A.M.) require less insulin to control blood glucose levels than the late morning hours. This increase in insulin resistance may be due to overnight hormonal activity.

The elevation in blood glucose levels seen during these hours is magnified when a person's insulin level declines or wears off in these morning hours. Therefore, the blood glucose level on awakening is often *not* the lowest during the night. Attempts to lower the prebreakfast blood glucose level can lead to unacceptably low blood glucose levels in the 2 to 4 A.M. time frame.

To avoid middle-of-the-night hypoglycemia:

1. Blood glucose should be monitored at bedtime.
2. Blood glucose should be monitored at approximately 2 to 3 A.M., especially (a) during attempts to lower prebreakfast blood glucose levels by increasing evening insulin doses; (b) when increased physical activity occurs during the day or evening; and (c) when decreased calories and/or carbohydrates were eaten.
3. Overnight lows may be prevented or avoided by increasing the bedtime snack (making sure that it is a complex snack, not just carbohydrate) if bedtime blood glucose is lower than 100 mg/dL, or there has been increased activity or decreased food intake.

Moving the evening dose of NPH from dinner (about 6 P.M.) to bedtime (about 10 P.M.) moves the insulin peak from the hours between about 2 and 4 A.M. (when insulin requirements are lower) to between 6 and 8 A.M. (when insulin requirements are higher, assuming peak levels at 8 to 10 hours after injection). This strategy recognizes the variations in nighttime insulin requirements and can help prevent middle-of-the-night lows while addressing prebreakfast highs. Another option is using Ultralente at dinner or bedtime, instead of NPH.

For many patients who use insulin pumps, the basal rate used during the first part of the night will be lower than that used for the period from 4 A.M. through breakfast. These rates are preprogrammed by the patients and are determined by their overnight and morning blood glucose levels. This multiple basal rate function of insulin infusion pumps makes them very helpful in dealing with the dawn phenomenon, especially when target prebreakfast blood glucose levels are not obtainable with usual injection routines.

Table 8.2. **Sick Day Management**

Goals
  Prevent hypoglycemia
  Prevent significant hyperglycemia
  Prevent ketosis
  Prevent DKA

Monitoring
  BG every 4 hr, or more frequently
  Urine ketones per void

Options
  Continue N, Lente, or U, and supplement R or lispro
  Lower N, Lente, or U by 20–50%, and supplement with R or lispro
  Discontinue N, Lente, or U; give R every 4 hr or lispro every 2–3 hr

Abbreviations: DKA = diabetic ketoacidosis; BG = blood glucose; N = NPH insulin; R = Regular insulin; U = Ultralente insulin.

In the Diabetes Control and Complications Trial, more than 50 percent of the severe hypoglycemic episodes occurred overnight. These occurred in patients using all regimens, even those with pumps. Prebreakfast blood glucose levels were often above target range. This emphasizes the need for overnight monitoring, a true awareness of the risk of overnight hypoglycemia, and the need to work to prevent this from occurring.

SICK DAY MANAGEMENT

Sick day management of children and teens with diabetes requires attention to detail and understanding of the many factors that contribute to metabolic control. The primary goals of sick day management are prevention and treatment of hypoglycemia, significant hyperglycemia, and ketosis; and prevention of diabetic ketoacidosis (table 8.2).

Sick day management should never be left to a child or teen alone. Parental supervision is essential, as is clinician availability. Not only must diabetes management be continued but the underlying illness must be diagnosed and treated. Illness and infection can present significant risk of deteriorating metabolic control in the child with diabetes because of two opposing effects:

> ➤ First, an increase in stress, or counterregulatory, hormones (cortisol and catecholamines) occurs during illness. These hormones have both hyperglycemic and lipolytic actions. They work against the action of in-

sulin, therefore producing a relative insulin deficiency and increasing the requirements for insulin.

➤ Second, during illnesses children and teens are often anorexic. The decrease in caloric intake that occurs with illness, especially when nausea and vomiting are present, causes a decrease in insulin requirements.

Such confounding factors make it easy to appreciate why even the most experienced families often need continuing consultation with the clinician for optimum sick day management. Here is what we tell the family to do when a child with diabetes gets sick:

ALWAYS GIVE INSULIN. A sick child or teenager always needs insulin but may need either more or less insulin than usual. You may be able to make insulin adjustments yourself, or you may want to call us for help.

ALWAYS CALL THE CLINICIAN WHEN

➤ moderate or large ketones are in the urine;

➤ small ketones occur through the day or on repeated mornings;

➤ vomiting occurs more than once;

➤ a cold, flu, fever, infection, or other childhood illness or injury affects blood sugar levels and/or causes ketones;

➤ a glucagon injection is given to treat low blood sugar, and/or vomiting occurs after a glucagon injection has been given.

Requirements for insulin during illness may increase, decrease, or remain the same. The signs and symptoms of the illness and of potential hypo- or hyperglycemia need to be sorted out. The basics of sick day management entail frequent blood glucose checks (at least every 4 hours), frequent urine ketone checks (each time the child urinates), and insulin adjustment (using Regular or lispro insulin) based on glucose levels and ketones. Trace ketones usually do not need adjustments, but moderate to large ketones require additional insulin.

When adjusting insulin doses, the options are:

➤ Continue the usual NPH or Lente dose, with Regular or lispro adjusted up or down, depending on blood glucose levels and/or urine ketones.

➤ Lower the NPH or Lente dose by 20 to 50 percent and supplement with Regular or lispro, the amount determined by blood glucose levels and ketones.

> ➤ Stop the longer-acting insulins and only give Regular, usually about every 4 hours, or lispro every 2 to 3 hours. This is the most flexible approach. Most children will need about 10 to 20 percent of the total 24-hour dose with each injection, including overnight. This also means that the child will require monitoring overnight.

Getting sick children to eat is often a major issue in managing diabetes. When a child is sick, it is more important than ever to have glucagon available in the home. If the ill child is unwilling or unable to take in solid foods, a parent can substitute similar calories of sugar-containing foods and beverages such as Popsicles, Jell-O, fruit juices, and non-diet sodas. Cases of persistent vomiting that prevent calories from being retained, or refusal or inability to take oral fluids or calories in any form, will require an emergency department or clinic visit. In most cases, the younger the child, the more urgent it is to get emergency treatment, because young children may become dehydrated quickly.

The following cases represent just a few of the sick day management challenges we have encountered.

CASE STUDY.   Maurice J., a 2½ year old, contracted a viral illness several months after being diagnosed with diabetes. He developed mouth blisters so severe that he could not eat or drink. His parents brought him to the local emergency department, where he was treated with intravenous fluids and insulin. After 6 hours, he still could not tolerate oral fluids, so he was admitted for 2 days for continuing treatment with intravenous fluids and insulin.

CASE STUDY.   Jordan H., aged 5 years, came down with a vomiting illness as 2 feet of snow piled up around his home. With the roads blocked by snow and the boy unable to keep even clear liquids in his stomach, Jordan's parents were afraid that the single glucagon kit they had would not be enough to get them through the blizzard. They were right. They used up the glucagon when Jordan's blood glucose dipped to 45 mg/dL, but 2 hours later, Jordan was still vomiting and the snow was still falling.

With Jordan wrapped in a blanket, his father carried him two blocks to the home of a neighbor who owned a four-wheel-drive vehicle and lived on a road that had been plowed. They drove Jordan to the local emergency department, where he was treated with intravenous glucose. He was discharged 6 hours later, when the vomiting had stopped and he had managed to retain some fluids. On leaving the hospital, the family refilled the glucagon prescription.

CASE STUDY.   Leslie S., aged 7 years, was diagnosed with diabetes when she was 5. She is 120 centimeters tall (46.8 in.), in the 50th percentile for her age; and weighs 20 kilograms (44 lb), in the 25th percentile. Her insulin dose is 6 units of NPH and 3 to 5 units of Regular at breakfast, 2 to 4 units of Regular at dinner, and 3 units of NPH at bedtime, for a total daily dose of 14 to 18 units. Her control is generally good, with glycohemoglobins that run about 7 to 8 percent (normal: 4.5 to 6.1%). She monitors her blood glucose levels three to four times a day and has had occasional mild to moderate lows but has never required glucagon.

One morning she woke up at about 6 A.M. and began vomiting. Her temperature was 105 degrees Fahrenheit, and her parents—having just gone through an identical illness with Leslie's older sister—anticipated that she would continue vomiting for several hours. Experienced with diabetes control, they did not give her the usual morning NPH. Based on the total of 16 units per day, Leslie's parents knew that she would need 1.5 to 3 units of Regular approximately every 4 hours while she continued to vomit. Exactly how much depended on her blood glucose. Her mother checked her blood glucose about an hour after she began vomiting, and it was 105 mg/dL, so she administered 1.5 units, along with some flat non-diet cola, a clear fluid. If the blood glucose had been 300, she might have used 3 units of insulin.

Leslie's mother monitored her blood glucose regularly every 2 to 4 hours and had glucagon available. She checked the child's urine ketones each time she urinated. The ketones increased to moderate but then cleared by evening. By dinnertime, Leslie had stopped vomiting but still had little appetite. Her parents urged her to eat, and she managed a slice of bread and a small bowl of chicken rice soup. Because of Leslie's decreased caloric intake, her mother decreased the bedtime dose of NPH to 1 unit, even though her blood glucose level had been in the mid-100s. Overnight, her blood glucose rose to 226 mg/dL, and it was 280 when Leslie awakened at 7 A.M. She felt much better, with her fever gone, no vomiting, and negative ketones. Her appetite returned, and she resumed her usual diabetes regimen.

DENTAL, MEDICAL, AND SURGICAL PROCEDURES

The basic principles of diabetes management which have been discussed throughout this book also apply to the specific contexts of dental, medical, and surgical procedures, with their unique needs. Here are a few basic guidelines that can help with management decisions.

First, even when a child is NPO (taking no oral food or drink), she still needs some insulin to remain metabolically normal. For the child or teen with Type 1 diabetes, at least some exogenous insulin is always necessary to avoid ketosis and hyperglycemia.

Second, if a medical, dental, or surgical procedure will require the child to be NPO for only a brief period, schedule the procedure for early in the morning. Since overnight is usually an NPO period anyway, scheduling a procedure for early morning poses the least disruption to the normal daily routine. (This is less of an issue for children and teens with insulin pumps.)

Third, taking into account the usual insulin regimen, the procedure that will be performed, and the length of the NPO period, an insulin regimen that works and is acceptable to the child, the family, and all involved clinicians should be determined collaboratively.

Fourth, blood glucose levels should be monitored every 1 to 2 hours, and urine ketones should be checked each time the child urinates. The insulin dose should be adjusted if blood glucose is outside the target range or ketones occur. In these situations, the upper end of the target range can be higher than usual (around 200 mg/dL), and the lower end should probably not go below 100. If the blood glucose is low, sugar should be given by mouth or, if the child is still NPO, intravenous glucose should be given. If the blood glucose is elevated or there are ketones, the amount of insulin given should be increased, using the child's usual sliding scale for Regular.

Insulin regimens for procedures are similar to those discussed above in sick day management. One frequently used regimen is to treat only with short-acting insulin. Another alternative is the basal-and-bolus regimen that children and teens with insulin pumps utilize. Think of the longer-acting insulins (NPH and Ultralente) as the basal dose, and the shorter-acting insulins (Regular and lispro) as the bolus. The basal dose works to keep the blood glucose in the target range when the child is fasting, while the bolus covers calories and carbohydrates consumed. Therefore, the basic principle is to continue the basal rate and omit or significantly decrease the bolus doses for the period when the child is not eating. For instance, if a child is on a regimen of Ultralente once or twice a day with Regular before meals, the Regular should be discontinued. The Ultralente may also need to be lowered, depending on the balance of the doses. For the child or teen on a more typical NPH and Regular or lispro regimen, one would likely lower the NPH and discontinue the Regular or lispro, although NPH does have a peak, not the more continuous steady level of Ultralente or the pump basal rate.

The cases of Peter and Carolyn illustrate how we apply these principles.

CASE STUDY.   Peter F., 11 years old, needed to have a number of teeth pulled to prepare for orthodontic work. His usual regimen was NPH and Regular at breakfast, Regular at dinner, and NPH at bedtime. His dental procedure was scheduled for the first thing in the morning. He took his usual evening NPH dose the night before and ate his customary bedtime snack. He took no insulin upon awakening. The procedure was completed by 9:30 A.M., and when it was over Peter took his usual morning NPH dose. Ninety minutes later he was feeling well enough to be a little hungry, and he ate some soft cereal and a milk shake, which he covered with his usual breakfast dose of Regular.

CASE STUDY.   Carolyn C. is 17 years old and has been successfully using an insulin pump for 2 years. She weighs 45 kilos (99 lb). Her current doses are 0.7 units per hour for basal coverage and 1 unit per 10 to 15 grams of carbohydrates for bolus doses. Her usual total daily dose is 30 to 35 units.

Carolyn needed to have all four wisdom teeth extracted. The 90-minute procedure was scheduled to begin at 8:30 A.M., and her dentist advised that as soon as it was completed, she would be able to take liquids and soft solids. Carolyn skipped her breakfast and her breakfast bolus and continued on her basal rate throughout the procedure. She checked her blood glucose every 1 to 2 hours, and when she began eating and drinking, she took her bolus dose based on her usual insulin-to-carbohydrate ratio.

On the morning of her procedure, Carolyn's blood glucose was 106 mg/dL when she woke, and it remained in the 80 to 150 range during the procedure. At 11 A.M. she had apple juice and a milk shake, with an estimated total of 30 grams of carbohydrates. She covered this with 3 units of Regular. During the remainder of the day, she had frequent small meals of pudding, yogurt, milk, or soft pasta, which she covered with her usual boluses.

Imagining a somewhat different course for Carolyn, one can sketch other possible scenarios and responses. Suppose she had awakened with her blood glucose level at 94 mg/dL but that it had risen to 158, 1 hour into the extraction procedure, and was up to 286 by the end, with ketones still negative. This is not unlikely, because of the effect of stress on blood glucose levels. Using the rule of 1,500, Carolyn could have divided her normal total dose (30 units) into 1,500, calculating that 1 unit of Regular would decrease her blood glucose about 50 mg/dL. Then a bolus of 3 units of Regular would have decreased her count from 286 to a healthy 150. If she was also planning to eat a snack containing 30 grams of carbohydrate, she would have taken another 3 units of Regular to cover it, for a total of 6 units.

In a third scenario, consider a situation in which, 1 hour into the procedure, her blood glucose decreased to 70 mg/dL. Since she was NPO, one treatment option would have been intravenous glucose, 5 percent dextrose at maintenance rate. If her blood glucose, rechecked in 30 minutes, showed no increase, the dextrose concentration could have been increased. Another possibility would have been to suspend pump insulin infusion for an hour, although she might still have needed IV glucose, since the effect of subcutaneous insulin does not stop instantaneously.

Another case to consider is that of a child on an insulin pump who has an emergency appendectomy. He will be NPO for an estimated 36 hours and on clear fluids for another 24 hours. Two choices for therapy are:

> ➤ Continue the basal rate of the pump, and as long as no calories are taken by mouth, give no bolus doses. Check ketones each time he urinates and blood glucose every 1 to 2 hours. Give IV fluids at maintenance rates, using 5 percent dextrose with electrolytes. Increase or decrease the basal rate if the blood glucose levels are outside the target range.

> ➤ Disconnect the pump and begin an intravenous infusion of Regular insulin. The usual dose is 0.02 to 0.05 units per kilogram of body weight per hour. Start maintenance IV fluids (5% dextrose with electrolytes). Check blood glucose and ketones and adjust insulin or IV dextrose as necessary. The goals for blood glucose would be 100 to 200 mg/dL, rather than the usual 70 to 120, with the higher target selected to avoid lows. Intravenous insulin has a lag time of minutes—as opposed to the hours-long lag time of subcutaneous Regular insulin—so this approach provides much closer control and more flexibility.

If a child or teen is to undergo a procedure that cannot be performed until afternoon and he must be NPO all day, IV glucose and low-dose IV insulin or small doses of subcutaneous Regular insulin will help to keep blood glucose levels in the target range.

9

Age-Specific Management

Most of the principles and strategies described throughout this book can be applied to managing diabetes in children of all ages. However, there are many issues that arise that are age-specific, requiring some insight into the child's developmental stage and his specific needs at this particular stage in life.

Handling these age-specific issues emphasizes the way in which the medical aspects of this disease interplay with the developmental issues of growing up and with every aspect of family life. No one knows better than the parent and the child himself what the individual child's needs are. Often the role of the clinician is as a consultant or adviser on age-related issues. The clinician and the family should talk together about these issues openly and on a continuing basis. While the following discussion is directed at clinicians, they may not always have a direct management role in the issues covered here. There are many times when this material may be useful to clinicians primarily as background, or as information to pass on to families.

INFANTS, TODDLERS, AND PRESCHOOLERS

It can be very frightening for the parents of a baby to learn that their child has diabetes. The tasks of management may seem daunting and disheartening. Many parents are terrified about the prospect of giving their tiny baby an injection, or even pricking her finger for monitoring.

Issues about feeding and eating on a schedule can be problematic with any baby, and the problems are compounded by the dietary supervision necessary to manage diabetes. It won't be easy to find a regimen that allows reasonable blood glucose control, avoids the lows that are so risky for babies, and permits a normal family life.

Because diabetes in babies is uncommon, it is hard to find other families to whom to turn for support. In the first weeks and months after diagnosis, the parents of a baby with diabetes will need close contact, support, and continuing reassurance from the health care provider.

True Type 1 diabetes is rare in babies. Less than 2 percent of all Type 1 diabetes is diagnosed in the first year of life. With another condition, transient diabetes of the newborn (TDNB), babies present with hyperglycemia, glycosuria, and dehydration. These infants are often emaciated, with an initial diagnosis of failure to thrive. The onset of TDNB, at a few days to a few weeks of age, can be sudden, and blood glucose levels may rise very rapidly. The condition is treated with tiny doses of insulin and usually resolves spontaneously, sometimes within a few days, with no residual effects, although some of these babies do go on to develop Type 1 diabetes later in childhood.

Type 1 diabetes can be very difficult to manage in babies for several reasons. Very young children often have erratic eating habits, with eating patterns that are irregular in both timing and quantity. Sleeping and waking times are also irregular, as is physical activity. And, of course, the child cannot describe symptoms.

The initial presentation of Cindy R. illustrates the difficulty of diagnosing a baby with diabetes.

> CASE STUDY.   Cindy R. was 15 months old when her parents realized that something was wrong. For several weeks her parents noticed that she was soaking through her diapers very quickly, to the point that they thought there was a problem with the absorbency of the current batch of diapers. Mrs. R. even thought about writing a letter of complaint to the diaper com-

pany. In addition, Cindy kept asking for drinks, holding out her bottle and pleading, "Drink, drink." When her parents noted weight loss and lethargy, they took Cindy to the pediatrician. Her blood glucose was 1,182 mg/dL. She was admitted to the hospital in ketoacidosis. Her ketones were large, and her electrolytes showed a bicarbonate of 9 mEq/L.

The crux of diabetes care for babies is that the parents (or some other adult caretaker) must do it all. This can be extremely difficult for many parents who find it painful to do something that hurts their child. Meanwhile, the child does not comprehend what is being done and has no cognitive framework to help him understand the frequent injections and finger-sticks. In some ways, these children may ultimately come to have a better understanding of the demands that a chronic disease makes on their everyday lives than children who are diagnosed at an older age, because they have never known life otherwise. Gradually they will be able to accept diabetes management as something they need to do every day, even though it may be inconvenient or uncomfortable. But these concepts cannot be explained to a baby.

A technical problem results from the tiny amounts of insulin that are needed for very small children. Insulin is marketed in 100-unit (per milliliter) vials, and the smallest syringes are marked in half units. A baby may need less than 0.5 unit per dose. It is possible to measure 0.25 unit, but less than that is imprecise for families and for clinicians. One alternative to this problem is diluted insulin, which can be prepared in the pharmacy, using diluent obtained from the manufacturer. Use of diluted insulin may lead to possible errors in dosage, and people using it must be vigilant, but it is necessary for the smallest babies. One way to dilute insulin for babies is to prepare the insulin as U-10 (1 part insulin to 9 parts diluent), so that 3 units in the syringe is actually 0.3 insulin units.

Often babies have a number of different caretakers: the mother and father, the grandparents, a daycare provider, a babysitter, even an older sibling. If diabetes care rotates among these caretakers, the potential exists for dosage errors or inconsistencies in amounts injected. It is usually helpful to decrease the number of caretakers giving injections to one or two. Other family members can assist in monitoring and providing food for the baby with diabetes.

Basic developmental feeding decisions—issues such as breast milk versus formula, and when to introduce solid foods—do not need to be influenced by diabetes. Young children with diabetes can be offered the same choices as children without diabetes. Growth must be closely monitored, as it should be for any baby.

There is no reason not to breast-feed a baby with diabetes, although this means that the baby's calorie consumption can only be estimated. Because of the difficulty of predicting how much a young child will eat and the need to avoid giving insulin that is not sufficiently covered by calories and carbohydrates, some parents of babies with diabetes wait until after feeding for the insulin injection. While this was necessary but not ideal using Regular insulin, the introduction of lispro makes this a satisfactory option.

The major medical goals of treatment for babies with diabetes are to avoid hypoglycemia, significant hyperglycemia, and ketosis. In infants, hypoglycemia is a much greater risk than hyperglycemia because of the potential for brain damage from low blood glucose and because a young child cannot tell you when he is feeling hypoglycemic. It can be very difficult to differentiate sleepiness and irritability from hypoglycemic symptoms without the child's own explanation of how he feels. Also, babies may have vomiting illnesses, which can progress to diabetic ketoacidosis.

Parents know their baby best and must pay close attention to symptoms. When in doubt, they should check blood glucose; and if it is impossible to check, they should assume that blood glucose is low. For babies, it is less dangerous to be high than low. Blood glucose goals are usually set higher in babies than in older children because of the risk of hypoglycemia. It is necessary to work hard to prevent lows and treat them quickly (e.g., with fruit juice, cake icing, or glucose gel) if they occur. Usually about 5 grams of glucose—about 1 to 2 ounces of apple juice or sugar-sweetened Kool Aid—is sufficient to treat a low. This should quickly be followed by something more substantial, either formula or breast milk or solid food, because the sugar alone will raise the blood glucose levels temporarily and will clear quickly.

Care must also be taken to prevent high blood glucose levels. While sucking continuously on bottles of milk or juice is discouraged for any baby, it is particularly bad for babies with diabetes, since it is difficult to cover with insulin and may cause consistently high blood glucose levels. Pacifiers can be used for babies who have a need for continual sucking.

Some parents find that the least traumatic time for injections is when the child is sleeping. This is fine, as long as the baby does not wake up crying when the injection is given. However, by the time the child has become verbal, we advise discussing injections during sleep in advance with the child and getting the child's approval.

Children sometimes become adept at the tasks of diabetes care at a surprisingly young age.

> **CASE STUDY.** Kevin L. was diagnosed at the age of 11 months. By the time he was 18 months old, his mother would say, "Okay, Kevin, time to check," and he would get his blood glucose meter, put it on the table for his mother, and hold out his finger to be stuck.

The same injection sites can be used for babies as for older children, and parents should pay close attention to which sites cause the child to become least upset when injected. Many children have marked preferences, and these should be followed as much as possible. In babies, it is sometimes easier to get a drop of blood for monitoring from a toe than from a finger, and this causes no short-term problems. However, we don't encourage getting into the habit of pricking toes because many people with diabetes have foot-related problems later in life. (See chapter 10.)

As children reach toddler and preschool age, it can be moving to see how their illness affects them, because there is still so much that they are too young to understand. Young Jason made a lasting impression on everyone on our treatment team.

> **CASE STUDY.** Jason T. was 4 years old and had diabetes for 2 years. At one clinic visit, he was very interested in telling us about his friend Scott, who had been ill with bacterial pneumonia and had been treated successfully with oral antibiotics. This made a big impression on Jason, who had become accustomed to his daily injections but still dreaded the procedure.
>
> Standing there, little Jason was eye-level with the sitting doctor, and he looked her straight in the eye. "Scott was a lot sicker than I am," he said, his lip trembling. "And he got better with pills. Couldn't I take pills for my diabetes?"

One issue that we think is important to discuss with parents of babies with diabetes is the matter of trust. Many parents find themselves grappling with this. Trust is important for a young child. She needs to get the sense that her life is safe and secure and that she can trust her parents and caregivers. It is important that the daily pattern of needles and finger-sticks doesn't compromise her trust. We tell parents not to lie to a child or cover up what is happening. It doesn't work to say, "This won't hurt," before an injection. The child quickly learns. It is better to say, "This will only hurt for a second, but then it will be fine." Tell the child, in a matter-of-fact way, "This will only take a couple of seconds," and "You need to do this to be healthy."

Parents must learn to keep the loving part of parenting separated from the diabetes part, at least momentarily. Don't cuddle the child and then surprise her with a shot; this can be very confusing. Surprise is never a good idea; consistency and quickness are. Some families find it helpful to have a separate place set aside for injections, so that the rest of the house is "safe." Parents should never be threatening about injections or use them as punishment. A comment such as "If you eat that candy, you'll have to get another shot" is not helpful.

Some children continue to scream before and during their injections. It helps if the caretakers are calm and matter-of-fact, but it can take time and a great deal of patience before this crying is resolved. See chapter 5 for further discussion about overcoming fear of injections.

Allowing the child who has a fear of injections to be manipulative about them will just make the situation worse the next time. A child may wheedle, "Just wait 10 minutes, and then I'll be ready," but in 10 minutes he will want another 10 minutes. It is important for parents to be firm. Again, the message is: "You need to do this to be healthy."

It is helpful to keep eating behavior as normal as possible for young children. Parents must be on guard against young children developing manipulative eating behavior and controlling the whole family's diet with their preferences. This is a situation in which giving the injection after eating can be very helpful, and in which lispro plays a useful role.

> CASE STUDY.   Keenan S. is 4 years old, and he loves Snickers bars. He has had diabetes for 1 year, and his parents allowed him to have one Snickers bar a week as part of his meal plan. This satisfied Keenan for a while, but after a few weeks, he began to demand more candy bars. His parents told him that they didn't think it was a very good idea. One evening, after Keenan's mother gave him his dinner insulin dose, he sat at the dinner table and refused to eat the meal. "I will only eat Snickers," Keenan announced. His parents said no and offered another alternative meal. Keenan continued to refuse to eat. Finally Mr. and Mrs. S., concerned that Keenan would become seriously hypoglycemic, gave in and allow him to have two Snickers bars instead of dinner. Over the next few weeks, Keenan's demanding behavior became a pattern.
>
> In order to resolve this problem, Keenan's parents told him that he could have only one Snickers bar every other day at dinner, and they stuck to it.

They changed their injection routine and began giving him his insulin after he ate. If he ate little, they gave him a minimal dose. After a few weeks, Keenan became more reasonable about eating, and the previous routine was resumed.

Insulin regimens for young children are similar to those for older children. One common regimen is two shots a day, each a combination of Regular or lispro and longer-acting NPH or Ultralente. Shots are usually given before breakfast and before dinner; in infants who are on only breast milk or formula, they are given about 12 hours apart. Regimens of three shots a day are also used (see chapter 6). Lispro is a very useful insulin for infants and young children; it can be given after a meal if needed.

Adults may sometimes have problems appreciating the concrete thinking of young children, the language they use, and what they understand and don't understand. Children often misinterpret what adults say. This can take their thinking in directions that adults would not anticipate.

> CASE STUDY. Every year the Juvenile Diabetes Foundation sponsors a "Walk for the Cure" fundraiser. Max J., who was 4 years old, had raised a great deal of money by signing up many sponsors among his relatives and neighbors. He successfully completed the walk around the zoo grounds, collected his pledges, and turned them in. Two weeks later, he said to his mother, "I did the walk, so where's the cure?"

This anecdote illustrates that children this young do not think abstractly. Adults need to continually remind themselves of this and make an effort to find out what their children are understanding. These are parenting issues, addressed by many books on parenting, but parenting becomes intertwined with medical care when one is treating children with diabetes. Clinicians should discuss these issues with parents, raising their awareness about their child's particular needs.

ELEMENTARY SCHOOL CHILDREN AND PRETEENS

We continue to be surprised at the young age at which some children can handle the tasks and responsibilities of managing diabetes.

> CASE STUDY. Heather and Megan R. are fraternal twins, aged 6 years. Heather was diagnosed with diabetes when she was 2; Megan does not have diabetes. One day in school, where the two girls were in the same

kindergarten class, Heather started becoming hypoglycemic. She was shaky and sweaty and seemed a little dazed. Megan was cool and unflustered; she'd seen this happen at home and knew what to do. "Heather needs sugar," she told her teacher matter-of-factly. The teacher got the juice that she kept in the classroom for Heather, and within 5 minutes after Heather had sipped the 4-ounce juice box, the shaky symptoms had subsided and she was able to participate in the class again.

Many young siblings of children with diabetes, like Megan, are capable of recognizing hypoglycemia and becoming involved in other ways, and they should not be left out of the management and care of the child with diabetes. When families come for appointments, siblings often come along at their own request to see for themselves what this aspect of diabetes treatment is all about. We encourage this.

Elementary school children and preteens, like younger children, may also have a different understanding of language and meanings than adults.

CASE STUDY.   Stephanie P., aged 8 years, told us in a clinic visit that she was having a hard time with monitoring. "As you practice, it will get easier for you to do," the nurse told her. "Practice!" Stephanie retorted. "This isn't practice, this is real life."

There are no reliable age guidelines that will determine when a child should or shouldn't be doing a specific task. It depends on the child's emotional maturation and willingness. We have 5 year olds who inject themselves, but children can inject before they are able to measure and draw up. As children begin to take over responsibility for their diabetes management, adult supervision must continue. Sometimes what seems to be maturity can be transient. Sometimes children will seem ready to assume a new task one week and shirk it the next. Sometimes life gets to be too much for children, and they just stop monitoring, or recording, or even giving injections, and "forget" to tell their parents.

Technical skills are likely to precede cognitive skills, and as children grow older their parents can talk to them about the thinking that lies behind the decisions that need to be made. Children must learn the problem-solving techniques that are necessary to handle the technical issues that might arise when they spend the night at a friend's house. They need to know, as they become involved with sports, the effects of exercise, and the fact that exercise may necessitate more frequent blood glucose monitoring. They need to learn to choose from a growing variety of foods.

As children move through the elementary school years, they begin to spend more and more time away from their parents. They are with their friends, their friends' parents, and other adults. Many children begin to spend nights away from home, with friends or relatives. They become increasingly competent to take over some of the self-care responsibility of diabetes and gradually learn the skills involved. This transition should take place in incremental steps. For blood glucose monitoring, for example, first let the child (like young Kevin, above) gather the supplies, while the parent continues to do the finger-stick. Soon the child can start sticking himself, and then recording the result. Again, it is important to emphasize the need for continuing adult supervision.

Children at this age are beginning to make more food choices, especially in school. Even if a parent packs a lunch, the child may trade food items or buy things. If the child is not part of food decisions, what is packed in the lunchbox and all the parent's well-intended food choices may end up not mattering. This means that children need the necessary nutritional education to make sound and healthy food choices.

Some families spend a lot of time planning around school lunch menus, which may change without warning. This can be a problem. There is a big difference in carbohydrate content between fish sticks, for example, and spaghetti, which is nearly all carbohydrates. The child has several choices in a situation like this. If spaghetti is on the lunch plate instead of fish sticks, she can just eat less. Or she can eat what she wants and exercise to make up for the additional carbohydrates, or take more insulin after school or at dinner. Another alternative, particularly for young children, is to just let the blood glucose be high for this period, although this is not ideal.

Children of elementary school age also begin to learn to recognize the signs of hypoglycemia. They must learn that they need to pay attention to these symptoms so that the low can be treated early. In the school setting, this takes a concerted effort of coordination among various people in the school, so that if a child begins feeling hypoglycemic, a system is in place for her to get sugar quickly. By the third or fourth grade, at the latest, a child should be able to keep glucose gel at her desk which she can take unobtrusively if she begins to feel low. All children with diabetes should have some sort of sugar substance on their person at all times to treat a low. It would be ideal if children were allowed to do their finger-sticking and glucose monitoring unobtrusively in the classroom, but many schools will not allow this because it is a process involving blood and sharp objects.

CASE STUDY.   Tyrone K., 6 years old and a first-grader, raised his hand in class and told his teacher that he felt low. The teacher told him to go to the nurse's office, where there were packets with different types of sugar products he could take. Tyrone set out on his own for the nurse's office and quickly became increasingly hypoglycemic—weak, shaky, and disoriented. He collapsed in the hall and was found a few minutes later lying face down on the floor. He was responsive, and was given glucose gel and then a small sandwich and juice.

As Tyrone's story illustrates, children should never be sent to the nurse's office alone. We have also heard of children who get to the nurse's office to find it locked, or cases in which a child is left alone in the office. This is risky. Also, children with diabetes should never be allowed to fall asleep in class.

Teachers, administrators, the school nurse, and any other involved school personnel must be notified in writing that a child has diabetes, and must be given an overview of the child's special needs and how to respond to these needs. This notification should come from the parents, and the required forms should be signed by the clinician. Other school situations where problems could occur are on the school bus, in the gym class, in any class with substitute teachers, and during afterschool activities. Again, it is important that the child always have sugar on his person and that a knowledgeable friend be on the bus or in the classroom with the child with diabetes. Most children are willing to let their friends know about their diabetes. The child with diabetes must understand that a knowledgeable friend on hand can not only assist with care but also be available in case of a low, to know what to do or to summon an adult for help.

The message for teachers, bus drivers, and anyone else involved in treating the child with diabetes is: *If in doubt, treat.* If the child acts strange or unusual—a normally well-behaved child who is irritable or grumpy, a child who bursts into tears, a child who is stumbling, a child who falls asleep in the classroom—give him some form of sugar. If he is not hypoglycemic, there are no long-term consequences of a little excess sugar. If he is hypoglycemic, a potentially dangerous situation has been averted. Whenever a child has had a suspected hypoglycemic episode during the school day, the parent should be notified.

Quick and appropriate handling of a child with diabetes in a large public school classroom is not always easy. Teachers may choose to have the child go to the nurse rather than to try to resolve a problem in the classroom. Even though this may be more disruptive for the child, it is often the only approach the school will allow.

Behavioral issues can also be a factor in the classroom, and it is not uncommon for children with diabetes to use their condition to try to manipulate a situation to their advantage. We see children use hypoglycemia as an excuse to get out of something—such as a test or a difficult assignment. Children may also act out because of problems that are occurring at home. Even though a problem has nothing to do with diabetes, it may be acted out in relation to diabetes, as Kathleen's case illustrates.

> **CASE STUDY.**   Kathleen V. was 10 years old, a fifth grader who had been diagnosed with diabetes the previous year. From the beginning of the school year, she was a frequent visitor to the nurse's office. She went to the nurse at least once a day, and sometimes three or four times a day, with a litany of complaints: "I feel sick." "I feel nauseous." "I feel high." "I feel low." Most of the time, during these visits, her blood glucose levels were in the target range. When we discovered this pattern, in the course of an interview with our nurse educator during a routine clinic visit, we encouraged the family to meet with a mental health counselor. They entered therapy, and as the problems—which eventually ended in separation for Kathleen's parents—were confronted and resolved, Kathleen made far fewer visits to the school nurse.

We encourage families to see mental health professionals in a variety of circumstances. While mental health and behavioral problems need to be considered in the context of the whole child and his medical concerns, primary care clinicians do not usually have the expertise or time necessary for sophisticated psychotherapy. Skilled primary care clinicians can do some initial mental health therapy, outlining the problem so that the family can begin to understand the issues. It is then useful to explain to them that comprehensive treatment can be provided by a competent and qualified mental health professional, and to refer them to such a practitioner when indicated. Henry and Tim were two patients who benefited from counseling. For further discussion of psychological issues, see chapter 11.

> **CASE STUDY.**   Henry L. was diagnosed with diabetes when he was 7 years old. He did well for a few years. However, as adolescence approached, he began having difficulties. He was unable to get beyond the fact of having diabetes. Every task necessary for diabetes management was always a chore for him. He didn't want his friends to know about his diabetes and kept his condition private. He was depressed, he stopped participating in

school and community activities, and he had few friends. Some children learn to control diabetes without the diabetes controlling them, but Henry couldn't seem to manage this. As he grew older, he felt that he couldn't go out because he needed to do injections and monitoring, that he couldn't eat out with his friends, and that he had no life beyond diabetes. We referred Henry for counseling, and as he matured and continued in therapy, he got better at handling some of the issues around his diabetes management. However, he still carries some anger, and his control is intermittent.

CASE STUDY.   Tim M., aged 12 years, was an intelligent child who knew what he needed to do for diabetes management but could not seem to follow through on performing the necessary tasks. He lacked the skills for handling adversity or responding situationally. "Is diabetes ruining your life?" the physician asked him during one clinic visit, and he answered promptly, "Yes." He seemed unable to handle simple changes in his routine. For example, he said that he wanted to eat a big snack after school but his current regimen wouldn't cover it. Just add a dose of Regular to cover the snack, we suggested, but thinking this through and executing it was too much for him to handle. So he would deny himself the snack and think about how diabetes was ruining his life, or else have the snack without covering it, and worry about how the high was affecting his health.

TEENAGERS

As children grow into their teenage years, we see many who weather adolescence well and handle diabetes management equally well. Others have a more difficult time. There is no question that a raft of new, complex, and difficult issues presents itself at this time in a young person's life. Diabetes, with its impact on so many of the activities of daily living, has an effect on many of these emerging issues.

Among the major things to be considered for teenagers with diabetes are the emotional and physical changes of puberty. Eating disorders tend to surface in adolescence. Risky and risk-taking behavior such as driving, drinking, cigarette smoking, drug use, and sexual activity become factors.

The shifting of responsibility from parent to child will be largely completed during the teen years. Just the simple question of who—if anyone—accompanies the teen to the medical visit can sometimes be a point of contention. It is necessary to work out compromises between the teen's need for privacy and the parent's need for knowledge. We find with our teenagers that it often works best for the clinician to examine the patient privately and talk with her about what she does and does not want to be discussed in her parents' presence.

Teenagers may feel conflicted about how much to tell friends about their medical condition, and who to tell. Should they tell someone on the first date? What about when they start driving? How about when they stay up late and go out for late-night snacks?

During puberty, insulin doses increase, not just because of the increase in body size but also because the hormones of puberty decrease insulin sensitivity, so that more units of insulin per kilogram of body weight are needed. Puberty and the adolescent growth spurt tend to increase insulin requirements by about 25 percent.

At the same time, there are health and developmental issues that are not related to diabetes, and these need to be sorted out. "Doctor, will you please tell him that because he has diabetes, he can't get a tattoo?" the mother of a 17-year-old patient pleaded. But we had to tell her that diabetes provides no medical reason not to get a tattoo.

Many other teenage issues do have a direct medical relation to diabetes care, however.

Driving

The rules for driving are no different for someone with diabetes than for people without diabetes. The driver has to be responsible not just for herself but for her friends in the car with her, and for everyone else on the road.

The consequences of hypoglycemia can be significant in someone who is driving, and it is often difficult to treat a low quickly while driving. We advise teenagers to monitor their blood glucose more frequently than usual when driving: before starting out on a trip, and at intervals, especially during a long drive. Drivers should have a low threshold for checking glucose and for ingesting sugar. They should be aware that it is easier for a low to creep up unnoticed when they are sitting and driving than when they are standing and walking around. They must have sugar-containing snacks in the car, strategically placed where they can be reached with one hand while driving—not in bubble wrap in the glove compartment or in the bottom of a purse. Keeping a tube of cake icing on the seat next to the driver, with the seal already broken, is a good idea. If a driver does feel that he is becoming hypoglycemic, he should pull over for a few minutes to have some sugar and wait until his blood glucose is normal before continuing to drive.

We begin talking to our teenaged patients about the responsibilities of driving when they are about 14 or 15 years old. It does not appear that individuals with diabetes have an increased risk of accidents. We are aware of only a few patients who have been in minor automobile accidents that may have been related to hypoglycemia. Some states require that diabetes be reported when a person gets a driver's license. When driving—as always—it is important that people with diabetes wear something on their person identifying them as an individual with diabetes.

Alcohol

The potential problems of teenagers and alcohol use cannot be ignored or overlooked. Statistics emphasize the necessity for confronting this subject head-on. According to the National High School Drug Use Survey by the University of Michigan's Survey Research Center, by the time they are in the 10th grade, nearly half of the teenagers surveyed reported having been drunk at least once, and more than 70 percent had tried alcohol. By the senior year of high school, that number rises to more than 80 percent who have tried alcohol and 60 percent who have been drunk.

Don't wait too long to address this subject. Perhaps the most sobering statistics are among younger teens. About 55 percent of eighth graders report some alcohol use, and more than one-quarter say that they have been drunk. These are 12 and 13 year olds. It is necessary to begin in early adolescence to talk to children with diabetes about drinking, to get a sense of their plans about drinking, and to explain to them the specific implications of drinking for a person with diabetes.

CASE STUDY.   Meredith R. is 17 years old, and she returned home at 1 a.m. from a party with her friends. Her parents watched as she tried to walk up the stairs but couldn't quite manage; her knees kept buckling and she dropped to the ground. She also seemed disoriented. Her parents had seen Meredith behave in a similar way when she was hypoglycemic. They checked her blood glucose and it was 128 mg/dL. Then they knew that her behavior was alcohol-related and had nothing to do with diabetes.

There are several physiologic effects of alcohol consumption that are particularly relevant to diabetes management. Alcohol can depress glucose release from the liver and therefore increase the risk of hypoglycemia. It also has a substantial number of calories—6 per gram—so that it adds calories to the daily intake, although it does not directly increase blood glucose. Working more like fat in the body, it can lead to weight gain.

Another problem for a person with diabetes who drinks is that when people drink they may tend to ignore what they're eating. The impairment of ability which is associated with alcohol consumption can lead to the development of unhealthy diabetes-related habits: forgetting to take insulin, forgetting to monitor blood glucose, and forgetting to eat. All of these can lead to poor blood glucose control as well as significant hypoglycemia.

A second problem for teens with diabetes who drink is the reverse of what happened with Meredith, above—the disoriented behavior that accompanies drunkenness can easily be confused with behaviors that result from low blood glucose, and the signs of hypoglycemia can be missed. Stumbling, falling asleep, confusion—is it alcohol or is it low blood glucose? Sometimes it may be both. This poses serious and real risks that should be known to teens with diabetes and their friends and families.

It is important to have a realistic attitude. We strongly discourage underage drinking, but we're not sticking our heads in the sand. We know that it happens, and that it happens frequently, as the statistics indicate. The following points should be emphasized when discussing drinking with teenagers with diabetes:

> Never skip meals or snacks when you drink. Alcohol will not directly raise blood glucose and should not be considered as a carbohydrate exchange.
> Drink only in moderation. Don't become so intoxicated that you don't know what's going on.
> Always wear diabetes identification. Bracelets or other tags can be purchased in a pharmacy or through organizations such as Medic Alert, whose brochures are often available in pharmacies or physicians' offices.
> Make sure that someone with you who is not drinking agrees to take responsibility for observing your behavior.
> Check blood glucose frequently.

Cigarette Smoking

Tobacco poses serious health risks to anyone who smokes. These are magnified for the person with diabetes. Smoking contributes to the risk of early vascular problems, which is already significant for the person with diabetes. The two risks together are compounded. The risks of atherosclerosis are discussed in detail in chapter 10.

It is necessary to begin counseling children at a very young age about cigarette smoking. We recommend introducing the subject by the time patients are 10 or 11 years old, asking them what their plans are concerning smoking. We try not to preach but just to give a realistic picture of the significant risks involved. If they are already smoking, we encourage them to get into a smoking cessation program as soon as possible. We also try to encourage smoking parents of children with diabetes to stop. Sometimes this is not very well accepted.

Sexual Maturation and Sexual Activity

Puberty increases insulin needs for both boys and girls. Girls must pay conscientious attention to their menstrual cycles because the monthly hormonal cycles may influence insulin need. Insulin requirements often go up in response to hormonal levels during the immediate premenstrual period and then drop when menstruation begins. A girl with diabetes should pay attention to what her body tells her about where she is in her cycle and connect this to her insulin needs, monitoring blood glucose levels even more frequently than usual during the premenstrual phase. Girls need to monitor and recognize premenstrual signs (e.g., breast tenderness, fluid retention, increased acne). Keeping good records will allow a girl to come up with a plan for the future and to be more proactive than reactive to the way in which changes in her cycle affect her insulin needs.

Sexual activity among teenagers is another fact of life that many adults would prefer to ignore. The many issues involved with teenage sex—emotional readiness, peer pressure, the risk of sexually transmitted diseases—are no different for teens with diabetes. Issues of sexual function usually do not occur in teenagers with diabetes, although such issues can become a real problem later in life (see the section on neuropathy in chapter 10). But pregnancy is the main issue that is specifically important for teenagers with diabetes.

Women with diabetes are at increased risk of giving birth to a child with a variety of clinical problems and/or birth defects. Pregnancies in women with diabetes are treated as high-risk pregnancies. Fetal malformations are related to the intrauterine environment in the woman with diabetes; their incidence is significantly decreased when the mother is in good control of her blood glucose. It is important for any woman with diabetes who is considering pregnancy to be in optimal control before conception. An accidental pregnancy, therefore, is particularly risky because control may not be optimal. This is why it is very important to emphasize the use of birth control and responsible sexual behavior for teenage girls with diabetes. We believe that pregnancies in teens with diabetes are best managed by a high-risk obstetrician.

Every day, women with good control of their diabetes have successful pregnancies and give birth to healthy babies. But it is important for teenage girls with diabetes to understand how significant the risks are for them and their babies. During pregnancy, a woman's insulin needs will vary, since hormonal activity in the first trimester enhances insulin activity, but glucose tolerance is reduced in the second and third trimesters. This means that meticulous monitoring is necessary; such monitoring can lead to very successful outcomes.

However, control that is less than optimal is associated with a range of defects and developmental problems in the baby, ranging from fetal death to congenital malformations to obesity and impaired intellect. Glucose is teratogenic, although the molecular mechanisms are not clear. Hyperglycemia in the early weeks of pregnancy is associated with a significantly increased risk of fetal malformation. A woman with diabetes has a two- to fourfold increased risk of giving birth to a baby with congenital malformations. The incidence of congenital heart disease is five times greater. Generalized myocardial hypertrophy, particularly of the intraventricular septum, is the most common abnormality seen in these babies. Caudal regression syndrome, a spectrum of defects involving the spine and lower extremities, is rare but strongly associated with mothers with diabetes.

Macrosomia in infants is also strongly associated with mothers with diabetes. Even pregnant women with tight control of their diabetes tend to give birth to larger than average babies, which is a reason for the increased risk of traumatic delivery or Caesarean section in pregnant women with diabetes.

In hyperglycemic mothers, glucose crosses the placenta, causing the fetal pancreas to produce extra insulin. This can result in hypoglycemia in the baby after birth. It can manifest in the form of seizures, lethargy, jitteriness, or poor feeding. If undetected and uncorrected, hypoglycemia can result in brain damage in the infant.

Other abnormalities that are associated with poorly controlled diabetes during pregnancy include respiratory distress syndrome, brain and neural anomalies such as anencephaly and spina bifida, and low calcium and magnesium levels in the first days of life. These low mineral levels are noted in approximately half the babies born to mothers with diabetes.

Illegal Drugs

Illegal drugs are unhealthy for a multitude of reasons. When parents sense that their teenagers are involved in significant risk-taking behavior, they should seriously consider counseling, not just for the teen but for the whole family.

We cannot ignore the reality of illicit drug use by teenagers. Findings by the Survey Research Center indicate that half of graduating high-school seniors have used illicit drugs. Marijuana, the most commonly used drug, tends to increase appetite, and teens with diabetes need to be aware of how excess calories will affect glucose control. Cocaine may reduce appetite and contribute to weight loss. All mind-altering drugs contribute to a lack of clear thinking and are likely to cause disruptions in the diabetes regimen which could lead to hypoglycemia or hyperglycemia.

10

Complications

Perhaps the most important thing to be said about complications is that they can be delayed and are likely preventable, at least to a large extent. Data from the Diabetes Control and Complications Trial (DCCT) demonstrate conclusively what most practitioners have suspected all along: that good control, with blood glucose levels and glycohemoglobins in or near the target range most of the time, will delay the onset and slow the progression of the most serious medical complications associated with Type 1 diabetes. Not only that, but for each decrement in glycohemoglobin levels there is an associated lowering of complication risk. The bottom line, the DCCT proved, is that control matters. Intensive control significantly lowered the frequency of eye, kidney, and nerve disease in people who didn't have these complications, and slowed the progression in those who did.

Complications for children and teens with diabetes can be thought of as acute, intermediate, or long-term. There are some complications that are primarily limited to children. This chapter discusses signs and symptoms of complications, how to moni-

tor for them, how to treat them, the understood etiology, and the risk factors that increase the likelihood of complications.
The acute complications of diabetes include

> ➤ hypoglycemia;
> ➤ hyperglycemia;
> ➤ ketosis; and
> ➤ diabetic ketoacidosis (DKA).

The intermediate complications include

> ➤ limited joint mobility, particularly in the hands;
> ➤ poor height and weight gain with delayed pubertal maturation;
> ➤ skin changes, primarily lipodystrophy; and
> ➤ necrobiosis lipoidica diabeticorum (NLD).

The long-term, chronic complications include

> ➤ retinopathy;
> ➤ nephropathy;
> ➤ neuropathy; and
> ➤ macrovascular disease, primarily atherosclerosis.

ACUTE COMPLICATIONS

Hypoglycemia

The most common acute complication of diabetes is caused by the
treatment, not the disease. The target range for blood glucose levels is
fairly narrow, without much flexibility in either direction. While hypoglycemia is rarely a cause of death, it is the most common reason that a
child with diabetes needs acute medical intervention and is a condition that
must be monitored for constantly and treated promptly. Fear of hypoglycemia, particularly after a severe hypoglycemic episode, can cause long-
term acceptance of unacceptably high blood glucose levels, which in turn
can lead to long-term chronic complications caused by chronic hyperglycemia.

It is difficult to set a specific limit that defines hypoglycemia, but most
clinicians agree that a blood glucose level below 60 mg/dL is too low. Some

people will have symptoms when their blood glucose falls below 70, although this is not common. But symptoms should always be heeded.

The immediate cause of hypoglycemia is too much insulin for the individual's needs at a given point in time. This may be because of insufficient food, too much exercise, or an insulin dose that was too high, either because an incorrect amount of insulin was given or because there was an error in planning what the dose should be. Hypoglycemia is a risk of tight control. The DCCT found that the incidence of severe hypoglycemia (requiring treatment by another person) was threefold higher in subjects in the intensively treated group. However, except in the case of young children, the benefits of tight control usually outweigh the risks.

Hypoglycemic symptoms vary from person to person and can be physical, mental, and/or emotional. The physical symptoms include trembling, dizziness, feelings of lightheadedness, increased pulse rate, heart palpitations, and sweating. These occur when the body's normal physiologic response to low blood glucose boosts the levels of the counterregulatory hormones. Epinephrine and glucagon are the early response, with cortisol and growth hormone in the second wave. Epinephrine is the normal stress hormone and is responsible for the fearful feelings that some people describe, and the pounding heart, trembling, and sweating. Other hypoglycemic symptoms are a response to the brain's being deprived of glucose. These symptoms can include visual disturbances (usually double vision), feelings of extreme hunger, headaches, stomach aches, and lethargy. A child can become very sleepy very quickly. He may stumble and move around clumsily. He may have trouble concentrating, feel dizzy or confused or disoriented, or respond inappropriately. Some people become very irritable, angry, and unreasonable and may resist treatment.

CASE STUDY.   Mark M., aged 20 years, who has had diabetes since he was 14, recognizes very specific symptoms of an incipient hypoglycemic episode. "My lips start to go numb, like too much novocaine," he says. "I sweat profusely, my hands start to shake, I get a little butterfly in my stomach. When I get that butterfly, I know it's time for me to have some sugar."

Mark catches 98 percent of his lows in plenty of time, but not 100 percent. He speaks of one period when he became lax in monitoring and missed or ignored low-grade hypoglycemic symptoms for a couple of weeks. "You get used to the feeling," he notes. "You stop recognizing the symptoms." At home with friends one evening, he became barely arousable, and his friends, not knowledgeable about diabetes care, put him to bed and left. He remembers waking to the taste of the chocolate mint ice cream his mother was spooning into his mouth, and learning that his blood glucose had dipped to 29. "I totally lost 4 hours of my life; I was completely out of it," Mark says. "That's pretty scary."

The standard treatment for hypoglycemia is to supply glucose, either directly (orally or intravenously) or indirectly (by the subcutaneous or intramuscular injection of glucagon). There is some risk in feeding a person who is barely conscious, as Mark was, because of the possibility of aspiration. Even putting glucose or cake icing in the cheek of a barely arousable child poses that risk, although many parents tell us that they do this.

The manner in which glucose must be supplied and the patient's ability to self-treat set up a continuum that describes the range of hypoglycemia, from mild to moderate to severe.

> *Mild.* The child or teenager is aware of what is happening, can express the low and seek appropriate help, and is able to take sugar orally.
> *Moderate.* The child does not recognize the low. This is seen more frequently in younger children. Another person detects the low, documents it, and treats it orally, with either liquid or solid food.
> *Severe.* The child cannot swallow, and the entire episode of treatment must be handled by another person. The child may experience seizures or coma. Usually glucagon must be injected or glucose must be administered intravenously.

Part of Mark's frightening experience was a phenomenon called hypoglycemic unawareness. Even after children are old enough to be able to sense hypoglycemic symptoms and attend to these symptoms themselves or notify someone, there are situations in which unawareness develops. Tight blood glucose control may lead to recurring hypoglycemia, and the feelings of the low may be so familiar to a person that he becomes less aware of these symptoms. The more lows a person has, the less awareness he may have of these lows, a dangerous cycle that may lead to even more significant hypoglycemia, as in Mark's case.

Hypoglycemic unawareness may be partly related to an impaired response of the counterregulatory hormones to the low blood glucose. When this occurs, the usual physical symptoms of a low do not occur or are minimal. A child may go very quickly from seeming fine to losing consciousness. Hypoglycemic unawareness is also related to frequent previous hypoglycemia and may increase with duration of diabetes. Several weeks of careful control with an emphasis on avoiding lows may reverse hypoglycemic unawareness.

The first line of defense against hypoglycemia is prevention. A person with diabetes should always have sugar on hand and glucagon readily available to quickly treat a low, but careful and frequent monitoring can go a long way to prevent lows from ever happening. Typically, we recommend that our patients monitor blood glucose levels four times a day, but a physically active child may want to check every 1 to 2 hours, depending on the intensity of the activity and the child's known personal risk of hypoglycemia. Monitoring is particularly important because symptoms are not always definitive. If a child detects a pattern of blood glucose dropping into the 50s every day before lunch, even though she does not feel low, she should recognize that she is at risk at that time of the day and make the appropriate adjustment—either lowering the morning insulin dose or eating more.

If the low is not averted, however, the treatment is usually quite simple and effective. The usual treatment for mild to moderate hypoglycemia is 10 to 15 grams of fast-acting carbohydrate (40 to 60 calories). This might be a sugar-sweetened soft drink, fruit juice, glucose tablets or gel, cake icing, or even a cup of milk (which contains about 12 g of carbohydrate). A candy bar is not usually recommended because there is often fat in the candy (e.g., in a chocolate bar) which slows down the glucose absorption and response.

The treatment dose should be adjusted for the child's size. Smaller children will need less. This can be tricky, and a number of factors must be considered. For example, where on the curve of insulin action is the low occurring? If the low occurs as insulin action is peaking, it could be that the blood glucose would rise on its own without treatment. If this is suspected, the child should be treated and the blood glucose level should be rechecked in about 15 minutes; if it has not risen above 60 to 70 mg/dL, the treatment should be repeated. Other variables to consider are the timing and content of the last meal, and exercise.

The response to orally administered glucose is not instantaneous. It may take 5 minutes, and it may take 15. Many patients have a tendency to keep eating until they feel better, but this can put them on a seesaw between highs and lows. One of the pitfalls of treating hypoglycemic episodes is overtreating. Experience will be instructive. We advise our patients to check their blood glucose a couple of hours after a low, and if the blood glucose level is high (e.g., above 180), they will know that they have overtreated and should scale back the next time.

In more severe instances of hypoglycemia, when the child or teen is vomiting or unconscious, it is necessary to administer glucagon. We recommend that anyone with diabetes have a glucagon emergency kit in her purse or pocket, at home, at school, at her grandparents' home, and wherever else she spends much time. Glucagon can be injected into a muscle or subcutaneously and begins working within minutes. The dose is the whole vial (1 mg), except for babies under 10 kilograms (22 lb), for whom half a vial (0.5 mg) should be used. If an unconscious child or teen does not quickly come around after a glucagon injection, or if the person providing the treatment is in any way uncertain, 911 should be called for emergency medical help.

Glucagon, like insulin, is a pancreatic hormone. Insulin works by storing calories. When there is an excess of insulin, the liver becomes filled with glycogen (stored complex glucose). Glucagon works to overcome this insulin effect and release the stored glycogen as glucose.

A problem with glucagon for some people is that it causes vomiting. When this occurs, a glucagon injection may need to be followed by intravenous glucose. Another difficulty with glucagon is that its effect peaks in about a half hour and clears quickly (within 2 hours), so that as soon as the child or teen is able, he should also eat or drink something that will raise blood glucose over a longer period.

We advise the parents of our patients not to be overly fearful about giving glucagon unnecessarily. Giving glucagon to a child who does not really need it will not cause any damage, just an elevation in blood glucose which will quickly come back down. After a severe low, it is usually prudent to decrease insulin doses.

Hyperglycemia and Ketosis

All people with diabetes have hyperglycemia to varying degrees, mild to moderate, virtually every day. This is part of life with diabetes and is related to imbalances between food, exercise, and insulin dosage. Learning how to prevent hyperglycemia is one of the major goals of diabetes management, and all people with diabetes are taught how to adjust their insulin doses to deal with varying blood glucose levels. In most cases this is accomplished with continuing adjustment of insulin doses, determined by patients, their families, and the management team.

The symptoms of hyperglycemia are described in chapter 2. In most cases, once diabetes has been diagnosed, hyperglycemia is detected by monitoring. Many children will know when they are high because of a frequent need for urination and increased thirst, symptoms that they may remember from the time of their diagnosis. Hyperglycemia may occur because the insulin dose was not sufficient when it was given, either because of inadequate dosing, missing a dose (or doses), consumption of excess calories, or not enough exercise.

Ketosis is indicated by positive urine (and sometimes serum) ketones, with no acidosis. There are no real symptoms of ketosis, except sometimes a fruity smell to the breath. Ketones, metabolites of fat, are the body's clue to insulin insufficiency. When the body begins to use fat stores for energy, ketones are formed. Because insulin is a very potent antilipolytic hormone, it takes a greater degree of insulin deficiency for ketosis to occur than for hyperglycemia to occur. This usually means that overeating can cause a person to become very hyperglycemic, with blood glucose levels in the many hundreds, but overeating by itself will not cause ketosis. Ketones are more likely to be formed in response to not taking insulin, not taking enough insulin, or having a significant illness.

Usually ketosis is accompanied by hyperglycemia. The exception is seen in the child with a vomiting illness, whose insulin dosage has been decreased because of lack of caloric intake. Ketones form in reaction to the relative insufficiency of insulin and the activity of the stress (counterregulatory) hormones, which are often elevated during illness and work to increase blood glucose and break down fat.

Ketosis is treated with doses of Regular or lispro insulin, usually an increase of 10 to 20 percent of the day's total insulin requirement. This is discussed in greater detail in chapter 8, in the section on sick day management.

Diabetic Ketoacidosis (DKA)

Diabetic ketoacidosis is a potentially life-threatening acute complication. It is the most common cause of death in young people (younger than the mid-20s) with Type 1 diabetes. The mortality rates from this complication have been reported to be as high as 6 to 10 percent. In other words, DKA is serious and should be treated with great care and attention. Prevention is the goal. Treatment of DKA should be provided by experienced personnel and should be administered where emergency care is prac-

Table 10.1.   **Diabetic Ketoacidosis Flow Sheet**

Feature	Monitoring Schedule
Clinical data Weight Vital signs State of consciousness	Onset of treatment and every 1–2 hr initially
Laboratory data Electrolytes (Na, K, Cl, HCO$_3$), venous pH	Every 1–2 hours for the first 4–8 hr, and then every 2–4 hr until DKA is cleared
Glucose	Hourly
Blood urea nitrogen, creatinine, calcium, phosphate levels	Every 4–8 hr depending on initial levels and type of fluids used
Urinary ketones and output (mL)	Every void
Fluids Potassium, phosphate, bicarbonate	Type and rate; record hourly input Record amounts added to fluid
Insulin	Dose, rate, and route

ticed—that is, in an emergency department, pediatric intensive care unit, or hospital floor where acute care is the norm. In our medical center, the emergency department physicians consult with the pediatric endocrinologist in cases of DKA. In other situations, the primary care physician may treat DKA. Meticulous monitoring of treatment parameters is mandatory and cannot be overemphasized. Use of a flow sheet greatly facilitates management, and one should be used (see table 10.1).

What Is DKA and How Does It Present?

Diabetic ketoacidosis can be defined as an elevated blood glucose (usually above 250 to 300 mg/dL) and the presence of ketonemia and acidosis (pH below 7.3, bicarbonate below 15 to 17 mEq/L). It can range from mild to severe. The occurrence of DKA in a child or teen with known diabetes is usually a failure of monitoring and early recognition.

The clinical signs and symptoms of DKA include polyuria, polydipsia, weight loss, the fruity breath odor of ketosis, nausea and vomiting, fatigue, and lethargy. Patients may be awake, drowsy, or comatose. Hyperventilation (the deep rapid breathing called Kussmaul respirations) and signs of dehydration (poor tissue turgor, dry mucosae, poor capillary refill, low

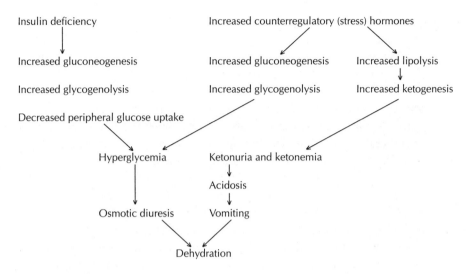

Fig. 10.1. Pathophysiology of diabetic ketoacidosis.

blood pressure and pulse rate, sunken eyes, and sunken anterior fontanelle in infants) may occur. Other findings at presentation can be abdominal pain and an elevated white blood cell count due solely to DKA.

What Causes DKA?

DKA is due to absolute or relative insulin deficiency along with elevation of counterregulatory (stress) hormones (catecholamines, glucagon, cortisol, and growth hormone). (See fig. 10.1.) These counterregulatory hormones work against insulin by increasing blood glucose levels (they increase glucose production and decrease glucose utilization) and increasing lipolysis. Combined with insulin deficiency, these hormonal abnormalities lead to hyperglycemia, lipolysis, and increased ketogenesis (increased acetoacetate and betahydroxybutyrate). An osmotic diuresis occurs due to hyperglycemia, producing dehydration. Electrolytes as well as water are lost through the kidneys. Ketones are produced as acids, leading to a decrease in blood buffers (bicarbonate). Compensatory respiratory alkalosis (hyperventilation or Kussmaul respirations) partially ameliorates this metabolic acidosis. Ketosis and acidosis lead to vomiting, which worsens dehydration. Electrolyte abnormalities occur in DKA due to intra- and extracellular shifts, vomiting, and urinary losses.

In children and teenagers with established diabetes, DKA may be caused by acute infections or vomiting illnesses, but omission of insulin is frequently the cause. This can be due to a misconception that when a child is ill and has decreased caloric intake or is nauseated and vomiting, insulin is not needed at all or is needed in much lower doses. It can also be due to deliberate omission. We see this in dysfunctional families, in which such omission may result from carelessness or from lack of supervision of a young child. Sometimes experimentation on the part of a teenager—for example, for weight loss—is the reason. It is believed that all or nearly all cases of recurrent DKA are caused by deliberate insulin omission, either by a child without the parent's knowledge, or even by the parent.

The degree of hyperglycemia in DKA often does not correlate with the degree of acidosis. Children and teenagers can be markedly acidotic (pH < 7.1, bicarbonate < 5 mEq/L) with only mild hyperglycemia (e.g., a blood glucose of 250 to 300 mg/dL). It is therefore important not to make any decisions about severity of DKA on the basis of the child's blood glucose level. The pH and bicarbonate levels must be determined.

Initial Assessment

The initial assessment of a child or teen with suspected DKA involves the following:

1. medical history and physical examination including
   a. vital signs
   b. body weight
   c. state of consciousness, i.e., mental status
   d. trigger(s) of this episode—for example, infection, emotional stress, insulin omission
   e. degree of dehydration, i.e., amount of weight loss, including signs of shock and poor perfusion
   f. signs of acidosis, i.e., vomiting, hyperventilation
2. laboratory tests
   a. blood glucose by meter—rapid result
   b. urine ketones by dipstick—rapid result
   c. blood gases (venous route is acceptable)
   d. blood glucose, electrolytes, blood urea nitrogen, creatinine, calcium, phosphate (or chemistry panel), and complete blood cell count with differential

3. a flow sheet for DKA treatment (the important factors to include are shown in table 10.1).

Principles of Treatment

There are several principles and goals of DKA treatment. Initially, clinical efforts must ensure adequate respiratory and circulatory function. Satisfactory support—for example, a modern emergency department or pediatric intensive care unit—must be available if needed.

The first line of treatment, therefore, is stabilization and correction of life-threatening problems, which may require fluid resuscitation for shock, or use of nasogastric tubes to prevent aspiration in comatose patients.

Next, the aims of DKA treatment are (1) to correct the fluid deficits, acidosis, and electrolyte abnormalities by careful rehydration, usually over 24 to 48 hours; (2) to give enough insulin to stop lipolysis and ketogenesis and to gradually lower the blood glucose level; (3) to monitor the progress of DKA treatment carefully to prevent (and treat if needed) the complications due to the treatment (e.g., hypoglycemia, hyper- and hypokalemia, hypocalcemia, cerebral edema); and (4) to identify and treat the cause(s) of the DKA episode (e.g., infection).

Specifics of DKA Treatment

The recommendations for the rate of fluid administration and the volumes of fluid to be used are the most variable in DKA management. The amounts of electrolytes, glucose, and insulin are generally agreed upon. Recommendations vary regarding the amount of the fluid resuscitation, and the total amount of fluid to be given in the first 24 hours, which is the time when the risk of cerebral edema (see below) is greatest.

The recommendations given here are the ones most generally agreed upon:

Fluid resuscitation. Give 10 to 20 milliliters of normal (isotonic) saline per kilogram of body weight during the first hour. Rarely, an additional bolus of 10 mL/kg will need to be repeated, as in the case of a severely dehydrated patient with persistent evidence of poor perfusion (delayed capillary refill and cool extremities, hypotension).

Next comes *replacement and rehydration.* This takes into account maintenance requirements (usually 1,500 to 2,000 mL/[m^2 × day]), replacement of the calculated fluid deficit, and replacement of ongoing losses, especially if they are excessive. If the patient's pre-DKA weight is known, accurate assessments of the deficit can be made. When this information is not available, a 10 percent fluid deficit is a reasonable estimate.

Fluid replacement can be given evenly over 24 to 36 hours. Slower replacement—for example, over 48 hours—should be given in those children with marked hyperosmolality or high calculated serum sodium levels (see the formulas below under "Sodium").

One can use a fluid rate in the range of 2,500 to 3,500 mL/(m² × day) for replacement and rehydration or calculate deficit and maintenance. It is best not to exceed 4 L/(m² × day), as in one study this was associated with an increased risk of cerebral edema. Occasionally, higher fluid rates are needed because of excessive ongoing losses (gastrointestinal and urinary), but this requires caution and especially careful monitoring.

During the replacement and rehydration period, the fluids given are usually half normal saline with added potassium and glucose (see below).

For patients with high corrected sodium and hyperosmolality, or a decreasing corrected sodium during treatment, a higher sodium concentration should be used—three-quarters normal or normal saline, along with slower replacement, over 48 hours, or perhaps longer.

While acidotic, the patient should be NPO. When the acidosis is cleared, the child can begin oral intake, perhaps with clear fluids first, but full meals can resume soon thereafter.

CASE STUDY. Bruce S. is 10 years old and has had diabetes for 6 years. When he came down with gastroenteritis, his insulin doses were decreased to almost nothing because of poor oral intake and vomiting. After 2 days he was in DKA. His parents noted the characteristic fruity odor and brought him to the emergency department. His usual pre-DKA weight had been 35 kilograms (77 lb), and his weight was now down to 32 kilograms (70 lb). Laboratory testing showed his blood glucose as 521 mg/dL, his pH as 7.16, and his bicarbonate as 10 mEq/L. His body surface area was 1 square meter.

Rehydration and replacement: replacement of a calculated deficit of 3,000 mL (35 − 32 kg) given over 1.5 days at a rate of 2,000 mL/day; plus a maintenance infusion of 1,500 mL/(m2 × day). This works out to a total daily infusion of 3,500 mL (2,000 + 1,500).

The IV was begun with one-half normal saline at 145 mL/hr (3,500 mL/24 hr), and potassium and glucose were added, as described below.

Sodium. Patients with DKA have lost sodium in their urine and have total body sodium loss. Because of hyperglycemia, the serum sodium level is artificially lowered by movement of water into the intravascular space. The measured serum sodium should rise as the blood glucose falls. The corrected serum sodium (determined according to the following formula) should stay steady during treatment. Paying attention to these points may lower the risk of the occurrence of cerebral edema. The formula for corrected serum sodium is

Corrected sodium = patient's serum sodium
+ [(patient's glucose − 100) ÷ 100] × 1.6

Example: If measured sodium (Na) = 130 and blood glucose = 600, corrected Na = 130 + [(600 − 100) ÷ 100] × 1.6 = 130 + 8.0 = 138.

The calculated osmolality should be normal (not low) during treatment:

Calculated osmolality = 2 (Na) + (glucose ÷ 18)

Example: If measured Na = 130 and blood glucose is 600 mg/dL, corrected osmolality = (130 × 2) + (600 ÷ 18) = 260 + 33 = 293.

Glucose. Glucose should be added to the IV fluids as the blood glucose drops to 250 mg/dL. Occasionally, it will need to be added earlier because of an excessively rapid decrease in blood glucose after the initial fluid resuscitation, once insulin has been started. Usually, 5 percent dextrose is added to the IV fluids; sometimes 7.5 percent and 10 percent will be needed.

Blood glucose levels should be monitored hourly. Use of a glucose meter provides instantaneous results. The IV glucose concentration should be adjusted up or down as needed to try to keep the blood glucose in the range of 150 to 250 mg/dL.

Potassium and phosphate. All patients with DKA have total body potassium loss, but their serum potassium level is variable—it may be normal, high, or low. Acidosis causes release of potassium ions from the cells. When insulin is begun, potassium moves back into the cells, and a decrease in serum potassium occurs.

Potassium should be added to the IV fluids after the initial fluid resuscitation as long as the patient is urinating and the serum potassium is not elevated. If hyperkalemia is present, potassium should not be added until the serum potassium has decreased into the normal range with insulin infusion.

If hypokalemia is present, potassium may be added earlier (during the initial fluid resuscitation) and requirements may exceed 40 mEq/L. Because both hypo- and hyperkalemia are potential causes of death, serum potassium must be monitored initially every 1 to 2 hours. Electrocardiogram rhythm strips can be helpful.

Usually, concentrations of 40 mEq/L are used. Potassium can be given in the form of the chloride, acetate, or phosphate salt. There are theoretical advantages and disadvantages to each salt. If hypophosphatemia is present, potassium phosphate is useful. The risks of phosphate administration are hypocalcemia and hypomagnesemia, so that a maximum amount of 1.5 mEq/(kg × day) of phosphate is reasonable. The use of 20 mEq/L potassium as potassium chloride and 20 mEq/L potassium as potassium phosphate (i.e., 40 mEq/L potassium—half as potassium chloride, half as potassium phosphate) is satisfactory for the first several hours of treatment. Calcium levels should be monitored when phosphate is given. Once the maximum phosphate has been given, a switch to all potassium chloride is satisfactory. Some centers prefer potassium acetate.

Bicarbonate. The use of bicarbonate in children has remained controversial. Most specialists agree that bicarbonate should be used only for severe DKA (e.g., pH less than 7.0) and that, if it is used, only a small partial correction should be attempted. The risks of bicarbonate are hypokalemia, hypernatremia, a metabolic alkalosis due to overtreatment, and a paradoxical cerebrospinal fluid and central nervous system acidosis. An infusion of 1 to 2 mEq/kg over a few hours can be given, again, only when severe acidosis is present.

Insulin. Continuous low-dose insulin infusion has been the method of choice for treating DKA for about two decades. Most physicians give a bolus dose of 0.1 unit per kilogram (U/kg) intravenously. Then, an infusion of 0.1 U/(kg × hr) is given. Regular insulin (not NPH, Lente, or Ultralente) is used. We prefer to give the insulin and the fluids through different IV fluid lines, so that the rates can be adjusted independently. Because of concerns about adherence of insulin to plastic tubing, about 50 milliliters of the insulin-containing fluid should be used to flush through the tubing before it is hooked up to the patient.

Most patients will respond very well to a dose of 0.1 U/(kg × hr). Rarely, there will be no improvement of acidosis after 2 to 3 hours; when that occurs, the insulin infusion rate can be increased by 50 percent, or it can be doubled. After the initial fluid resuscitation in the first hour of DKA treatment, when blood glucose may fall significantly, insulin should lower the blood glucose level by about 50 to 100 mg/(dL × hr). If the level drops more quickly, it may be necessary to add glucose (5% dextrose) to the IV fluids.

The acidosis will be corrected more slowly than the hyperglycemia. Therefore, when the blood glucose decreases to about 250 mg/dL and acidosis is still present, glucose should be added to the IV fluids. The glucose should initially be in the form of 5 percent dextrose, which should be increased to 7.5 percent or 10 percent if necessary. It is preferable not to reduce the insulin infusion rate when the patient is still acidotic. However, if absolutely needed, the rate can be decreased by 25 to 50 percent (e.g., to between 0.075 and 0.050 U/[kg × hr]). Once the acidosis has been corrected, the IV insulin rate can be decreased further.

How and when to stop the insulin drip. We usually continue the IV insulin until the child or teen is alert and taking oral fluids well without vomiting or nausea, the acidosis is corrected (pH is normal, bicarbonate is greater than 18 mEq/L), and urine ketones are, at most, trace to small. It is preferable to give the first dose of subcutaneous insulin before a meal. The insulin drip should continue until 30 to 60 minutes after the first subcutaneous dose.

CASE STUDY.   Brittany Q. is a 13-year-old postpubertal girl who has had diabetes for 5 years. Her usual weight is 55 kilograms (121 lb). She developed DKA after skipping several days of insulin injections in an effort to lose weight. She was not monitoring ketones and therefore did not detect the onset of ketosis. She did not tell her parents that she was sick until after 8 hours of vomiting. She was brought to the emergency department at 8 P.M. Her weight at that time was 50 kilograms (110 lb), representing a 9 percent loss. Initial laboratory tests showed blood glucose at 653 mg/dL, a pH of 7.12, and a bicarbonate of 7 mEq/L. Brittany was awake but sleepy. After the initial fluid resuscitation, she received a 5-unit IV bolus of regular insulin, and then a 5 U/hr IV drip was started (after the tubing was flushed with about 50 milliliters of the insulin infusate).

Brittany's recovery was uneventful. She was kept NPO for the treatment period. By 4 P.M. the next day, she was no longer acidotic; her blood glucose was down to 212 mg/dL, and she had a pH of 7.42, a bicarbonate of 22 mEq/L, and trace ketones in her urine. She continued on the insulin drip. At 5:30 P.M., Brittany received her usual evening dose of 8 units of Regular and 12 units of NPH. Dinner was served at 6:00 P.M., and the IV insulin infusion was discontinued between 6:00 and 6:30 P.M.

Here is a variation of the above case: At 3 A.M., the patient was no longer acidotic and had a blood glucose of 176 mg/dL, normal pH and bicarbonate readings, and negative urine ketones. It would have been acceptable to give her subcutaneous insulin at 3 A.M., with a small snack and the IV insulin infusion discontinued 30 to 60 minutes later. However, in order to stick to her usual dosing pattern, the IV insulin infusion was continued at a 25 percent reduction, and her glucose-containing IV fluids were also continued for a few more hours. At 7 A.M. she received her usual morning insulin dose of 15 units of Regular and 25 units of NPH. Breakfast was served at 7:30 A.M., and the IV insulin drip was discontinued between 7:30 and 8:00 A.M.

The IV insulin infusion can be continued until a normal mealtime in order to get back on the child's usual schedule promptly. This is similar to the plans used to treat and monitor diabetes during medical, dental, and surgical procedures.

If the patient is newly diagnosed with diabetes, or if for some reason there is no information about usual insulin doses, subcutaneous insulin can be started in several ways. First, give 0.1 to 0.25 U/kg of Regular before a meal, assess the response, and continue to give premeal Regular for a few meals. Don't forget the need for overnight coverage. A dose of Regular at 6 P.M. won't last until 7 A.M. the next day. Once you have a sense of the dose requirement, switch to the anticipated outpatient regimen, for instance, Regular and NPH twice a day. Second, estimate the daily requirements on the basis of age, pubertal status, and body weight, and start regular and NPH subcutaneously before breakfast or before dinner. The dose details are discussed in chapter 6.

Cerebral edema. Cerebral edema is a uniformly feared complication of DKA and its treatment. Unfortunately for pediatric practitioners, it occurs primarily in children. It is unexpected, unpredictable, and often fatal, and entails significant cognitive morbidity in those who survive it. Even when careful attention has been paid to all the details of DKA management as discussed above, cerebral edema can occur and produce rapid neurologic decompensation. On occasion, other central nervous system insults, such as hemorrhage or thrombosis, occur during DKA. Cerebral edema is the cause of about one-third to one-half of DKA-associated deaths in children.

There is no clear and accepted cause of cerebral edema. A number of hypotheses or factors have been suggested: (1) an overly rapid fall in blood glucose or a drop in blood glucose to a level that is too low; (2) excessive fluid administration—too much, too soon; (3) the use of fluids that are hypotonic; (4) the use of bicarbonate in DKA treatment; and (5) failure of the serum sodium to increase as the blood glucose drops with treatment, indicating an excess of free water administration.

Close monitoring of treatment factors and of the child, clinically, are therefore very important. The indications that cerebral edema may be occurring include severe headache, fluctuating or worsening mental status or behavior changes, pupil changes (dilated, sluggish, unequal or fixed), the onset of hypertension or hypotension and bradycardia, and problems with temperature regulation.

If cerebral edema is suspected, treatment should be given: specifically, IV mannitol (about 1 g/kg of body weight or small doses repeated hourly), intubation and hyperventilation, and fluid restriction. Consultation and monitoring in an ICU with an intensivist and neurologist or neurosurgeon should be done promptly. Even with early and rapid treatment, the morbidity and mortality are significant. Therefore, prevention of DKA is the goal.

INTERMEDIATE COMPLICATIONS

The intermediate complications of Type 1 diabetes include a number of miscellaneous problems, some of which involve growth and development and are specific to the pediatric population.

Growth Impairment

The majority of children and adolescents who are in fairly good control of their diabetes grow normally with no growth impairment. This can be seen in growth chart after growth chart of children with diabetes. However, both undertreatment and overtreatment with insulin can result in growth abnormalities. Even subtle decreases in rates of height and weight gain should be noted, and treatment strategies should be quickly re-evaluated when this occurs.

Chronic undertreatment with insulin is associated with poor weight gain, poor linear growth, delayed skeletal maturation (bone age), and delayed pubertal maturation. The degree of growth impairment can be significant in children with poor management. It is therefore very important to obtain careful height and weight measurements at every examination, to plot height and weight on growth charts, and to look closely for any deviation from standard patterns.

Conversely, excess insulin tends to be associated with excessive weight gain. Weight gain may be associated with tight control, an association that clinicians have observed and that the DCCT results validated.

In some patients, particularly adolescent girls, clinicians have observed a tendency not to cover food with insulin in order to avoid weight gain. This can be a great temptation for overweight young people, since it is presumably easier than dieting; if the behavior is repetitive, it should be considered an eating disorder.

> CASE STUDY.   Nancy S., a 16 year old, went to a high school for the arts, played the piano, and wanted to become an actress. However, she was too overweight for the acting roles she wanted. She started using her diabetes to control her weight and was in a state of chronic ketosis, although not acidosis. She would spill ketones but knew how to take just enough insulin to prevent acidosis. She kept her weight moderate but never got as thin as she would have liked.
>
> "Don't you feel bad physically, being so out of control?" we asked Nancy at a clinic visit. "I'm not out of control," she answered, "I'm in a controlled high." We explained to Nancy that she was paving the way for long-term, serious, life-shortening complications, but she had a fatalistic response. "I'm going to die young anyway," she told us. We referred Nancy to a specialist in eating disorders.

Short-term growth delay is usually reversible; however, if growth problems remain undetected and untreated late into adolescence, there may be permanent consequences. Delayed puberty and delay in skeletal maturation are part of the same pattern of insulin insufficiency as poor linear growth and poor weight gain. Mauriac's syndrome, also known as diabetic dwarfism, is severe growth failure associated with chronic inadequate insulin treatment. Children with the disorder are very short, with slow growth, very delayed skeletal maturation, and a pot-bellied appearance because of liver enlargement. Mauriac's syndrome has been rare in the United States since the advent of modern monitoring techniques and is associated with extremely high glycohemoglobin levels.

Mauriac's syndrome is the most extreme of the growth disorders that are related to diabetes. A less severe—and more common—growth disorder is seen in the case of Ted H., who was profiled in chapter 4. Despite having been diagnosed with diabetes at age 6, Ted had not received medical attention through adolescence and had very poor glycemic control. As he began paying closer attention to insulin dosage and monitoring, his growth rate increased, and he moved from far below the 5th percentile back up to the 5th percentile in height and weight.

Limited Joint Mobility

Limited joint mobility (LJM) is seen occasionally in the pediatric age group with Type 1 diabetes and is most likely associated with longstanding poor control. Modern monitoring and glycohemoglobin measurement make this complication less common today, but LJM should be looked for periodically, especially in teens. The way to diagnose it is to have the child put her hands together in a praying position, or flat horizontally, or vertically against a hard surface. If she cannot get her fingers down flat, she has LJM. This disorder is associated with other long-term complications, primarily because it is associated with poor glycemic control.

Limited joint mobility is believed to be caused by glycosylation of connective tissue proteins because of longstanding hyperglycemia. In our experience, it is uncommon. Most of the children and teens with LJM whom we have seen also have a history of multiple episodes of DKA and persistently high glycohemoglobin levels. It is a marker for poor control. Some children will notice joint stiffening, but more often the clinician has to look for it.

Limited joint mobility begins in the outer digits, the metacarpophalangeal and proximal interphalangeal joints, and can progress to the larger joints. The only treatment is improved glycemic control.

Lipodystrophy

Lipoatrophy (thinning) and lipohypertrophy (thickening) are local skin problems that can be caused by insulin injections. With the highly purified human insulins that have been used for the past decade, lipoatrophy has become very uncommon. A site where lipoatrophy has occurred looks like a crater; it is a painless indentation where the skin surface remains normal but the subcutaneous fat has atrophied. If this does occur, the site should not be used for injections, or injections should just be made around the edges.

Lipohypertrophy is thickening of subcutaneous fat and is much more common. The most likely causes are improper injection technique (particularly improper injection depth) or always injecting in the same spot. Lipohypertrophy presents two problems: there may be delayed or irregular absorption of insulin from hypertrophic sites, and the lumpy spots may be unsightly.

Repeated use of the same injection site causes these obvious physical complications, yet we see patients with these problems again and again. Reluctance to adequately rotate injection sites is a common issue for children and teens with diabetes. Sometimes the repeated use of a site can result in anesthesia at the site, so that the child will prefer it for injections. The clinician should examine injection sites at every visit, not just looking at them but feeling them; if there is thickening at a certain spot, that spot should be avoided.

> CASE STUDY. Gary W. was diagnosed with diabetes at 9 months of age. As a baby and toddler, he hated injections and would scream and shriek and try to run away. As he got older, he would hide from his mother at injection time. It was very hard on the family, and Gary would only tolerate shots in his arms. By age 2½, Gary had developed lumps on his lateral upper arms, which he would show off to us on his clinic visits as if they were big muscles. As a young child he continued to refuse to use other sites, and his parents injected around the edges of the hypertrophied sites. As he got older, he was persuaded to sometimes use his legs as injection sites, but he also developed lumps on his legs.

Some children may be more prone than others to lipohypertrophy. However, Gary's problem may have been caused by his unwillingness to do sufficient site rotation.

Insulin Allergy

True insulin allergy is very unusual. When it does occur, we recommend consultation with an immunologist or allergist, and desensitizations may be necessary. Insulin allergy manifests with hives at injection sites and/or with systemic hives. Local hives are not uncommon and are not usually significant. If they occur, the first step, if the patient is not on human insulin, is to switch to human insulin. If the symptoms occur systemically, treatment with insulin, which is necessary for life, becomes a major problem and may require formal desensitization.

Necrobiosis Lipoidica Diabeticorum

Necrobiosis lipoidica diabeticorum (NLD) is a skin manifestation that occurs primarily in females. Seen predominately on the shins, it appears in the form of shiny atrophic areas and can lead to skin breakdown, ulcerations, or infection. It is very uncommon, diagnosed in 0.3 percent of diabetes patients. Sometimes it is observed before diabetes is diagnosed and suggests that the clinician should check for diabetes. Its etiology is unclear, but because it is sometimes seen before diagnosis, it is not associated with long-term hyperglycemia.

Cataracts

Cataracts are also uncommon in children and teens with diabetes, but they do occur and are another reason for looking carefully at patients' eyes. Hyperglycemia causes the lens to pull water in, and thus high blood glucose alone can cause temporarily blurred vision. "Sugar cataracts" are thought to be the result of an abnormality in the osmotic mechanism in the lens. These cataracts often occur after an episode of DKA and resolve as the blood glucose is brought down. If blurriness continues when sugar is normalized, it is important to consult with an ophthalmologist. Another form of cataract, "juvenile cataract," is the result of the metabolism of glucose to sorbitol in the lens and may need surgical removal.

Impaired Intellectual Development

There are data to support the theory that abnormalities in learning occur in individuals when they are hypoglycemic, but this is very difficult to assess. Sophisticated cognitive testing demonstrates that hypoglycemia is associated with decreased performance. What is not clear is if hypoglycemia causes any permanent impairment. Some studies have found that children who develop diabetes before the age of 5 years have diminished cognitive development, compared to healthy siblings. This is believed to be related to hypoglycemia.

It should be emphasized that it is by no means a given that a child with diabetes will have intellectual impairment. Many clinicians have patients who were diagnosed before the age of 4 years and who are on the dean's lists at Ivy League colleges. Clearly, many people with an early diagnosis of diabetes achieve the same levels of intellectual accomplishment as people without diabetes.

Associated Autoimmune Disease

Since diabetes is itself an autoimmune disease, it is associated with certain other autoimmune diseases. The most common of these is autoimmune thyroid disease, which occurs in two forms: hyperthyroidism, which is uncommon; and hypothyroidism, which is more common. Hypothyroidism is seen in as many as 15 percent of children and teens with diabetes. All children and teens with diabetes should be screened for thyroid function. The screening should include thyroid antibodies and thyroid-stimulating hormone (TSH) levels. We generally screen at the time of diagnosis, and if antibodies are negative at that time, we repeat the screening every couple of years after diagnosis. If antibodies are positive, we follow with rechecks for TSH at least every year. It is important to be aware of the signs and symptoms of thyroid dysfunction.

The symptoms of hyperthyroidism are goiter (enlarged thyroid gland); proptosis (protruding eyes); weight loss; increased pulse rate; increased systolic blood pressure with decreased diastolic blood pressure; diarrhea and increased frequency of stools; increased appetite without weight gain; jitteriness; poor sleeping; increased energy; and heat intolerance.

The symptoms of hypothyroidism are goiter; dry skin; constipation; slow linear growth with increased weight gain; delayed skeletal maturation; delayed dental maturation; lethargy; and cold intolerance.

Lack of normal linear growth in children with diabetes may be due either to poor diabetes control or to associated hypothyroidism. These conditions are usually fairly simple to distinguish. First, children who have poor linear growth due to poor diabetes control will not be gaining weight, unlike the child with hypothyroidism, who will gain weight but will have slow linear growth. Second, laboratory tests (for glycohemoglobin, thyroxine, and TSH) allow rapid differentiation of these problems.

Hypothyroidism is fairly easy to control; hyperthyroidism is more difficult. Antithyroid drugs such as propylthiouracil (PTU) and methimazole are used to treat hyperthyroidism. Hypothyroidism is treated by replacing l-thyroxine, and there are several synthetic thyroid hormone products on the market.

Other associated autoimmune endocrine diseases are rare and primarily include Addison's disease, which is autoimmune adrenal insufficiency; and pernicious anemia, or vitamin B_{12} insufficiency. In our clinic we do not routinely screen for these diseases unless the family history is positive for them or the child also has thyroid disease. If there is a positive family history or any symptoms, the clinician should have a low threshold for screening. The symptoms of Addison's disease include weakness, electrolyte abnormalities, increased skin pigmentation, poor tolerance of infections, fatigue, and lack of adequate weight gain, and can progress to adrenal crisis. The symptoms of pernicious anemia include sore tongue, general weakness, numbness and tingling in the extremities, and jaundiced skin color.

CHRONIC LONG-TERM COMPLICATIONS

The organs and systems most commonly affected by chronic long-term complications in diabetes are the eyes (retinopathy); the kidneys (nephropathy); the peripheral nerves and the autonomic nervous system (neuropathy); and the cardiovascular system (macrovascular disease—primarily coronary artery disease, which leads to myocardial ischemia and infarct; cerebral vascular disease, which leads to stroke; and peripheral vascular disease, which leads to ulcers and amputations).

Most children and teens with diabetes do not experience these chronic complications, which usually do not develop until people are well into adulthood. However, some early symptoms are observable in childhood, and some children do develop full-blown complications.

CASE STUDIES.   Malcolm H. was diagnosed with diabetes at age 2. Denise W. was diagnosed with diabetes at age 5. They have fairly similar histories. Both had many (more than 50) episodes of DKA and longstanding poor control. They had missed many insulin doses. We first saw Malcolm when he was 14 and Denise when she was 15. Both had background retinopathy, hypertension, and gross proteinuria. Denise also had limited joint mobility.

There is general agreement that chronic hyperglycemia causes long-term complications. Several mechanisms may affect the changes that lead to complications. One theory centers on abnormalities in the polyol-myoinositol pathway and the conversion of glucose to sorbitol, a sugar alcohol, by the enzyme aldose reductase. In a hyperglycemic condition, aldose reductase causes an accumulation of sorbitol. A subsequent series of biochemical processes has been shown to be important in the formation of cataracts and in diabetic neuropathy. These findings have led to the experimental use of a number of drugs that inhibit aldose reductase to see if they prevent disease, but none is yet available commercially. This research is ongoing.

A second proposed mechanism focuses on the fact that in a state of chronic hyperglycemia, glucose binds to proteins, including connective tissue protein such as collagen, changing the properties of these proteins. A chain of chemical reactions ends in the accumulation of glycosylation end products, which remain indefinitely in the body. Researchers are also investigating this avenue. Studies of one drug, aminoguanidine, which inhibits the glycosylation of proteins and the cross-linking of these end products, show promise.

There is also a series of risk factors that are known to influence the likelihood of developing long-term complications. Some of these are under people's control and therefore must be aggressively heeded. The first is blood glucose control, the issue that has been discussed throughout this book. Other risk factors include cigarette smoking, high blood pressure, and elevated blood lipids (cholesterol and triglycerides). High protein intake may also contribute to nephropathy. Smoking increases the risk of vascular problems by narrowing blood vessels, and restricted blood flow can cause cells to die. This can lead to heart and coronary artery disease, impotence, and amputation. Young people with diabetes should be aware of these direct consequences of smoking, the potentially devastating impact of compounding hyperglycemia with the effects of smoking, and the importance of smoking cessation. Likewise, elevated lipids and hypertension should also be treated.

There are probably also genetic components to the development of complications. Not every patient with poor control develops complications, and some with good control do. These genetic components are not well understood.

Retinopathy

Some form of diabetic retinopathy is seen in most patients with insulin-dependent diabetes. However, as the DCCT conclusively demonstrated, good glycemic control is associated with decreased incidence and slower progression of retinopathy. The 125 adolescents in the trial's intensive therapy group experienced 50 percent delay in the onset of clinically significant retinopathy, compared to the control group. In addition to glycemic control, hypertension is also a risk factor for retinopathy.

Background retinopathy causes changes in the retina, but these changes do not affect vision. Eighty to 90 percent of patients who have had Type 1 diabetes for 15 to 20 years eventually develop some degree of background retinopathy. Proliferative retinopathy is more serious and may cause retinal detachment and lead to vision impairment. Diabetes is the underlying cause of approximately 10 to 20 percent of all cases of blindness and is the single most frequent cause of blindness in U.S. adults.

However, vision problems are not inevitable for the person with diabetes. Only 5 to 10 percent of people with Type 1 diabetes become blind. Laser therapy is extremely effective in treating certain proliferative changes. Again, the key is vigilant monitoring and early detection. It is important to follow patients regularly and to treat laser-treatable lesions immediately when they occur. Macular edema, with fluid leakage from the macula, also decreases vision and is not unusual in people with diabetes. It can be treated with laser photocoagulation, and the vision decrease is reversible if caught early enough.

Meticulous ophthalmologic care is a critical part of diabetes management. All people with diabetes should be followed regularly by an ophthalmologist or an experienced optometrist, one who is familiar with the special needs of people with diabetes. Significant retinopathy is rare before puberty. Current recommendations are that every child with diabetes aged 10 years or older should have an initial comprehensive dilated eye examination within 3 to 5 years after diagnosis, followed by annual examinations. Prior to the age of 10 years, eye examinations are rarely needed. In addition, the primary care or diabetes clinician can do routine fundoscopic examinations yearly.

Background Retinopathy

Microaneurysms or dot hemorrhages may be seen in a comprehensive ophthalmologic examination but do not appear to affect vision or cause any observable symptoms. It is also not clear that they necessarily progress to proliferative retinopathy. Background retinopathy usually manifests initially with microaneurysms, small outpouchings of blood vessels. These can sometimes be seen by the non-ophthalmologist but are best detected with sophisticated testing. Fluorescein angiography is very sensitive in finding vascular leakage and microaneurysms. Fundus photographs are also recommended. Use of these two techniques has been found to detect background retinopathy 2 years earlier than conventional ophthalmologic examination.

A comprehensive eye examination will also detect hard exudates, whitish or yellowish regions on the retina. These may progress to soft exudates and then to venous changes, as background retinopathy worsens. These changes still do not affect vision. Intraretinal microvascular abnormalities (IRMAs), in which blood vessels start growing within the retina, and not out into the vitreous, may also develop. This is considered a preproliferative change.

Proliferative Retinopathy

Proliferative retinopathy is defined as new vessels and fibrosis growing into the macula and vitreous of the eye. The exact mechanism of proliferative retinopathy is not fully understood, but it is believed that the narrowing of blood vessels that results in insufficient blood supply to parts of the retina triggers the oxygen-deprived retina to manufacture a factor that creates new blood vessels. These are unstable and may bleed. The bleeding causes proliferation of fibrous tissues, which can pull the retina away from the eye, resulting in a detached retina. Although a detached retina can sometimes be surgically corrected, it can be very difficult to reattach a detached retina that is bound up with fibrous tissue.

Nephropathy

Diabetic nephropathy is a leading cause of end-stage renal disease. Approximately 30 to 40 percent of patients with Type 1 diabetes will eventually develop end-stage renal disease (ESRD) and will need dialysis or transplantation or both. A pre-DCCT study determined that in a person with diabetes, macroproteinuria was found to develop an average of 10 to 15 years after diagnosis, and renal failure occurred an average of 20 years after diagnosis.

Kidney enlargement is noted early in most people with Type 1 diabetes. The glomerular filtration rate (GFR) and renal blood flow are increased, and there is an associated increase in kidney size and weight. Over time, there is thickening of the capillary basement membrane in the glomerulus and expansion of the mesangium, the tissue around the glomerulus, eventually resulting in glomerulosclerosis. This can lead to progressive renal insufficiency, characterized by increasing serum creatinine and urea nitrogen and decreasing GFR.

Microalbuminuria, the development of a small amount of albumin in the urine, is the initial clinical finding indicating nephropathy and precedes the development of clinically significant kidney damage. Microalbuminuria is related to duration of disease and to glycemic control and is rare in prepubertal children. It is a signal that something abnormal is occurring, and it should be heeded. Initially, the microalbuminuria may be intermittent, but then it is likely to become persistent.

As the DCCT and other findings indicate, there is a growing body of evidence showing that increased GFR can be normalized by improving blood glucose control. As with retinopathy, attentive and aggressive monitoring translates to prevention. Kidney function should be monitored after 5 years of disease or at the onset of puberty. This means annual urinary microalbumin tests. We use timed overnight urine collections, which our patients can collect at home, reporting the start time and end time to us. Spot urine collections can also be used. Clearly, any patient who has a dipstick showing positive protein needs to have more sensitive analysis done. Microalbuminuria occurs before the urine dipstick becomes positive for protein, and is a more sensitive indicator.

We have found it useful to obtain baseline microalbumin levels in the first year after diagnosis, and we generally obtain these levels yearly. There is no definitive general agreement about what level of microalbumin is considered significant. Most clinicians will consider levels above approximately 30 micrograms per minute (μg/min) to be elevated. Urine albumin that is greater than 200 to 300 mg/day (equivalent to 140 to 210 μg/min), is considered to be significant gross proteinuria. Once a person's urinary albumin is in the high range or hypertension accompanies microalbuminuria, the GFR will begin to drop, leading to progressive renal insufficiency.

Hypertension is a very significant risk factor for nephropathy and is an important part of screening for this complication. Blood pressure should be monitored accurately at each clinic visit, several times a year. Hypertension should be treated aggressively using an angiotensin-converting enzyme (ACE) inhibitor, with the goal of lowering the blood pressure to at least the 90th percentile for the patient's age.

When there is significant urinary albumin (greater than 200 to 300 mg/day), ACE inhibitors are recommended, even in the absence of hypertension. There is some difference of opinion among clinicians about the use of ACE inhibitors when urinary albumin is between 50 and 200 mg/day and there is no hypertension, but many are treating in this range. Anyone being considered for treatment with ACE inhibitors should be seen by a nephrologist.

In preventing nephropathy, it is also important to address other risk factors, including glycemic control. Cigarette smoking has been shown to be another important factor in the development of nephropathy. Diet may be another factor; low-protein diets are believed to slow the progression of diabetic nephropathy in adults with diabetes. However, protein restriction for children may have negative effects on growth and should only be undertaken with caution and careful growth monitoring.

Sometimes the proteinuria can be so significant that a clinical picture similar to nephrotic syndrome develops. The patient will lose so much albumin through urine that blood protein drops, osmotic pressure in the blood decreases, and considerable edema results.

One reason that we have found it useful to have baseline overnight urine microalbumin levels in the first year after diagnosis is that some children who do not have diabetes have a condition called orthostatic proteinuria, in which they spill protein during the day but not at night when supine. Knowing this early can be helpful. Sometimes a kidney biopsy is necessary to determine definitively whether there are diabetic changes in the kidney.

> CASE STUDY.   Amy M., who is 14 years old, is on an insulin pump and has excellent glycemic control and a normal blood pressure. Several years ago she showed evidence of orthostatic proteinuria. A fractionated 24-hour urine specimen found that she spilled protein during the day but not overnight. A nephrology consultant recommended biopsy, which was done when Amy was 11 years old, 4 years after her diabetes diagnosis. The biopsy was normal, with no diabetic nephropathy.

Neuropathy

Symptomatic neuropathy is uncommon in children and teenagers with diabetes, although studies using nerve conduction velocities detect subtle nerve changes after 4 to 5 years of the disease. Neuropathy eventually occurs in about 50 percent of people with Type 1 diabetes, and it is related to duration of disease and to the severity of hyperglycemia. It is caused by abnormalities in the polyol pathway. Improvements in glycemic control can help to lower the risk of neuropathy.

Subclinical neuropathy in children with diabetes has been described. One monitors for this by checking ankle reflexes (deep tendon reflexes) and pressing a tuning fork against the child's toes and ankles, to see if she can feel the vibrations. Another test is to have the child close her eyes as we touch a monofilament to various parts of her feet. If she has protective sensation, she will feel the light touch, but loss of that sensation is an early sign of neuropathy.

The most common form of peripheral diabetic neuropathy is bilateral and symmetrical sensory neuropathy. Its symptoms are loss of reflexes, numbness, pain, paresthesia, and sometimes hyperesthesia. It most often occurs in the legs and feet but can also affect the hands. It often starts at the toes and progresses upwards. Peripheral diabetic neuropathy is usually associated with poor control and improves with better control. Good foot care should start in childhood, because once sensation is lost, injury can occur without the child being aware of it, as one teen found out on the beach.

> CASE STUDY.   Jasmine J. is 18 years old and has had diabetes for 12 years. One hot summer day, she spent a great deal of time walking barefoot on the sand at the beach. At the end of the day she noted that the soles of her feet were extensively blistered from the hot sand, although she had been unable to feel herself being burned.

A wide variety of other neuropathic conditions can also affect people with diabetes. These can include problems with single motor nerves or with the spinal root.

Autonomic neuropathy is rarely seen in children or teenagers. It can manifest as delayed gastric emptying, diarrhea, orthostatic hypotension, poor bladder emptying, and some changes in cardiac reflexes such as reduced heart rate variability during breathing. Impotence is another form of autonomic neuropathy for which men with diabetes are at significant risk as they grow older. A study reported in *Diabetes Care* in February 1996 found erectile dysfunction at an overall rate of 20 percent in men over the age of 21 who had had diabetes for more than 10 years and took insulin. This only affected 1.1 percent of men under 30 years of age with diabetes, but by age 43 the rate had risen to 46.1 percent. Impotence is associated with other complications such as severe eye disease and elevated glycohemoglobin, suggesting that tighter blood glucose control is preventive.

Macrovascular Disease

The rate of macrovascular disease, early hardening of the arteries, is increased in people with diabetes, although, again, this complication is very rare in children and teenagers. Macrovascular disease includes coronary artery disease, peripheral vascular disease, and cerebrovascular disease. It is a major mortality factor for adults with diabetes, who have increased and early coronary artery disease, leading to heart attacks and strokes. In adult women, the considerable protection that estrogen provides against atherosclerosis is obliterated by diabetes. However, control of the risk factors—hyperglycemia and elevated lipids—clearly has a preventive effect, as the DCCT confirmed.

In the child or teen with diabetes, just as in their peers without the disease, the major means of preventing macrovascular disease is a prudent diet that is low in fat, particularly in saturated fat. Lipids should be screened regularly. We do a total lipid profile upon diagnosis, after glucose control has been established. If levels are borderline or abnormal, they are repeated and evaluated. People with consistently elevated lipids should be considered for drug therapy, as new treatments become increasingly available. For patients with normal levels, we repeat the lipid profile periodically. Recommendations are every 5 years. The levels should be compared to age-appropriate normal ranges. Other risk factors, including family history, hypertension, and smoking, must also be addressed.

11

Psychological Issues

A s has been emphasized throughout this book, many of the medical and dietary issues of diabetes are closely intertwined with psychological issues. There are many fears and concerns that children and teenagers and their families have in relation to diabetes. Chief among them are the following:

➤ They are concerned that the diagnosis of diabetes requires significant lifestyle changes and commitments, particularly with regard to organization, planning, and food issues.

➤ Diabetes has both acute and chronic complications that many people fear. This includes the daily risk of hypoglycemia, as well as anxieties and dread about long-term complications. Parents are very concerned about these issues, although children themselves often exhibit the typical childhood sense of invulnerability.

➤ Parents and children fear that the treatment for diabetes—injections and monitoring—hurts.

- ➤ The child or adolescent perceives himself as having a defect that will make him unattractive to friends or less desirable for dating or marriage.
- ➤ Diabetes is relentless, and you can never take a real vacation from it. Many times each day, the child and family must deal with decisions that affect diabetes management and therefore the child's health and, ultimately, life.
- ➤ People often act as if blood glucose monitoring results and glycohemoglobin counts are report card grades and they are being judged on the basis of these readings. Who is doing the judging—their parents? the children and teens themselves? health care providers? Often it is the patients themselves.
- ➤ Young children may think that they have been bad and that diabetes is their punishment. This belief can be very pervasive and deeply felt and is often not fully recognized.
- ➤ Despite the family's best efforts, the risk of complications is still uncertain.
- ➤ Having a chronic disease exacerbates all the child-caring tasks that have to be dealt with as any child grows up, and it complicates the task of becoming independent.

The above list includes concerns that are specific to diabetes. Psychological considerations revolving around more general health care issues are also intertwined with diabetes management. Health-related behaviors, knowledge, and skills are impacted by individual and family functioning. A broad range of psychosocial issues will end up influencing diabetes management and adherence to treatment requirements. These include expectations and attitudes about health care; past experiences with illnesses and health care personnel; goals for treatment, which can range from specific to general and which change with time; moods; personality traits (e.g., extroversion or introversion); and sources of significant stress in the family, such as death, divorce, other illnesses, or financial concerns. Don't underestimate financial problems. Job loss, job security, debt, and health insurance are extremely important in many families and can end up having a significant impact on diabetes management.

Diabetes is a family disease, and the family must work together with the health care team to solve problems. Families, including siblings, need to develop plans to share diabetes-related tasks. Good communication and cooperation are essential. All family members should be able to discuss their feelings about diabetes in an open and nonjudgmental way.

Since psychological issues are so intertwined with all the other aspects of diabetes management, the primary care clinician needs an understanding of these issues within every patient's family. An early gauge of psychological adjustment will be the way in which the child and family accept the diagnosis of diabetes, and their willingness to learn about diabetes, take all of the necessary knowledge steps (of which there are many), and begin changing behaviors.

CHANGING BEHAVIORS

The clinician can assess whether the family is willing to make the necessary behavioral changes for effective diabetes management by considering a number of questions. How are they reacting emotionally to some of the issues important in diabetes management, such as fears about injections, fears about hypoglycemia, and fears about long-term complications? Who are the key support people in the patient's life? Is there any psychiatric illness in the family? What are the body weight goals for the patient? How do the patient and/or family see diabetes affecting body weight and attractiveness? Eating disorders and depression have been shown to impact negatively on glycemic control.

The way in which the patient and family interact with the various health care providers—either the primary care clinician or the specialist and various members of the team—is also important. Patients and their families must feel free to ask questions; the clinician must take the time to explain what he or she is doing, and why. The clinician must be constantly vigilant, not to criticize but to question and be available for problem solving.

The medical setting should provide a sense of support and security even in the darkest hours. Providing psychologically oriented health care—care that enables patients to have trust in the provider's availability and willingness to be there even when they are despairing, feeling frustration, and overwhelmingly burdened by this disease—is an important part of diabetes treatment. Patients need this safe place that the clinician can give them, especially since no one can tell them, "If you do A, B, and C, your disease will be cured," or even assure them that "if you do A, B, and C, you will be free of complications."

Cultural factors may influence the way in which a family perceives the meaning of illness and its treatment. Some people see illness as a punishment. They may think that God is punishing them and that they must have done something bad to deserve this disease. Some stricter religious beliefs may foster this perspective. Another attitude that may be culturally related is a fatalistic approach, a sense that there is nothing that can be done to change the outcome of this disease. Of course, as has been emphasized in every section of this book, such an attitude toward the management of diabetes could not be further from the truth.

In treating patients with diabetes, many clinicians will encounter people with poor learning skills and ability. It may be years before they can master the tasks of diabetes; they may never fully master them. We recall one case of a single mother of five children who could not read or do any math. In a situation such as this, it is necessary to simplify the regimen as much as possible. For example, the patient's mother could be instructed to use pre-mixed NPH and Regular insulin, the clinician can put a piece of tape on the syringe at the dose level insulin should be drawn to, and identify morning doses with a picture of the sun and evening doses with a picture of the stars. And the clinician should be aware that this child's diabetes will never be under as tight control as that of someone on a multiple-shot regimen who is able to make the many decisions that are required every day to maintain such a regimen.

It is important to be aware of all these issues for every child and teenager who has diabetes. It becomes particularly important when people are not meeting all their goals in treatment, and when you get a sense from patients and families that the disease is overwhelming them.

Clinicians should not be reluctant to refer patients and families for mental health services if the family perceives that psychosocial or behavioral issues are interfering with the achievement of desired goals. We always recommend psychological counseling for patients who can't meet the medical goals of treatment or who seem to have personality or psychological barriers to successful management.

Our suggestion is not always heeded. For instance, in the case of a child who can't get over the blow of having a chronic disease, we will strongly recommend therapy, but if he is not motivated to seek psychological help, he can't be forced to do so. There are some patients you may not be able to help, but you should never give up. You never know when a circumstance will occur which will push someone into making a change. We recall a teenage patient who had turned a deaf ear to our advice about the association of tight glycemic control and prevention of complications. But she was somehow struck by a public service announcement she had heard on television about how diabetes causes blindness. She had heard this dozens of times from her parents and health care team, but when it came from a different source, it triggered a new awareness. She recognized herself, saw her ability to have some control over her condition, and began to take the appropriate steps.

A collaborative relationship is necessary among clinicians and patients and their families. As has been repeatedly emphasized, this is a disease of home- and self-management, and all must be full partners. Patients and families need to participate actively in setting treatment goals and agendas. Much of the work that clinicians do concerns diabetes knowledge, diabetes skills, and health behaviors, because this directly affects glycemic control, and glycemic control—along with other risk factors (e.g., smoking)—affects long-term complications. However, it is clear that one also needs to think about how to contribute to diabetes knowledge, skills, and health behaviors at a deeper level by influencing family and individual functioning. Underlying factors such as depression and eating disorders should be pursued and treated. Maintaining and improving the therapeutic alliance between the family and the health care provider should be a continuing effort.

An internally set goal is usually much more achievable than one that is externally imposed. Clinicians should be realistic about the choice of goals. We can say to a child, "We want you to monitor your blood glucose five times a day and write your numbers down and fax them to this office once a week." But if this interferes with the child's own goals, and he wants to monitor only twice a day, he will seldom do what we ask. However, the clinician should convey to him that he must also be realistic in setting his goals. Monitoring twice a day might be acceptable, but monitoring twice a week certainly would not be.

Ask children and teenagers about hidden concerns. Be specific. Ask them what they are worried about. You'll hear responses such as these:

➢ "I'm worried that I'm going to have a hypoglycemic reaction while I'm driving, so I'll eat candy before I get into the car, and then I worry about that."
➢ "I'm worried about my new boyfriend seeing me take a shot, so I won't carry insulin or glucagon or syringes with me. I won't even tell him about glucagon, and I make sure my blood glucose is running in the 200s or higher when I go out with him."

> "I worry about getting stuck somewhere without any insulin or any food. Like getting separated from my mother at the mall."

> "I don't want the kids in my class to know I have diabetes, because they'd tease me and wouldn't pick me for their sports team. If they know I have diabetes, I'll be the last kid picked."

The hurt from these rejections, and perceived rejections, can stay with a child for many years. Even if it's not important to play the game, it is still important to be accepted, to be picked for the team. The feelings engendered by these situations, and their relation (or perceived relation) to diabetes, will become intertwined with a child's feelings about her disease and its impact on her life.

ANGER, GUILT, AND HOPE

It is not always easy for children and teenagers to honestly communicate their feelings. It is often easier for younger children, particularly when they are given a little bit of encouragement and a sympathetic ear. "I'll bet you're really angry at having diabetes," we will say to them, or "What's the hardest thing about this for you?" Sometimes it will help a child just to yell, "I hate diabetes!" and this should be allowed and encouraged. Or suggest a pillow or punching bag labeled "diabetes," which a child can pound when he is angry.

Sometimes, some of these negative feelings and worries will manifest themselves in the form of anger at the clinician. The health care provider has a different perspective from the family. We see these children all the time, we usually know what we should do for them, their problems are everyday occurrences for us, and we will go home at the end of the day. But they may think that their lives are falling down around them and will never be normal again.

The child's (or parent's) anger should be addressed in an empathic way. Acknowledge it, acknowledge that it is real and reasonable, and don't try to minimize it. Talk about what the underlying fears and worries are. Listen carefully. Health care providers often think that they are in the role of providing the answers. In fact, this is what clinicians have been trained to do. But this may sometimes lead to trying to solve problems that are out of our purview, rather than helping an individual figure out how to solve his own problem. It might seem easier to propose a solution, but first ask the patient or parent: How do you think this problem can be resolved? What are your ideas? If he can think of no potential solutions, then propose a number of solutions to choose from. This is an important form of empowerment.

One subtle indication of anger at the clinician is a common response one might get when asking for input from patients—the remark, "Well, you're the doctor." This abdication of responsibility, turning the burden of the disease over to the doctor, can be an expression of resentment and underlying hostility directed at the health care professional, who, after all, sometimes might seem like the bad guy to a confused and unhappy child or a frightened and overwhelmed parent. We have some families who believe that because they come for treatment at a major medical center, we should be able to cure their child's diabetes.

Anger at the disease may be expressed in seemingly trivial ways. Parents get angry if they have to wait to see the clinician, if they can't find a parking place, if the person drawing blood has to stick the child more than once. This is anger at the disease which is redirected toward the clinician. You have to recognize this, be tolerant of it, allow the negative feelings, and allow the anger to be expressed. It is very important for the clinician to respond in a compassionate way. Try not to take negative feelings personally. Most negative feelings are about the disease and life with the disease, not about you. Most are surmountable.

Guilt is also a common feeling, especially among parents and older children. Parents—particularly parents who also have diabetes or have a family history of diabetes, and thus have a sense that the genetic predisposition came from them—may think that the fact that their child has the disease is their fault. Guilt can be powerful. "I did something wrong when I was pregnant," a mother will think. Or "I fed my child the wrong foods or allowed her to eat something she shouldn't have." When the parents are well educated, an empathic clinician can usually dispel these feelings with accurate information, but sometimes misconceptions linger. In families with lower educational levels, dispelling the guilt can be very difficult. Cultural background may also influence this.

Parents and health care providers should have similar goals in approaching children with diabetes. Their role is to keep hope alive (a phrase that is borrowed from the title of a book about psychotherapy)—for patients, for families, and perhaps for ourselves—and to facilitate a normal life. If the only goal in a child's life is keeping her blood glucose in good control, then she doesn't have much of a life. Managing chronic disease gets very tedious—and for no one more so than the patient. There are various ways to keep hope alive, and sometimes just small acts or activities such as the following can change a child's focus and renew hope:

➤ Set aside 1 day a week when the parent gives injections and takes care of monitoring.
➤ Come up with creative suggestions for food treats—for example, pretzels, Goldfish and other kinds of crackers, animal crackers, and vegetables and fruits cut into unusual shapes.
➤ Award points for successfully fulfilling the tasks of diabetes care and reward accumulations of points with "prizes"—family activities such as a camping trip, a movie, a dinner at a favorite restaurant, or a trip to the arcade. A teen might want to use points for items of clothing. (Note that points are awarded for carrying out tasks, *not* for the results of monitoring.)

CASE STUDY.   Jennifer M. is 8 years old and comes to our clinic from a town about 150 miles away. She is a very good-natured and motivated child, with highly motivated parents, and they all work very hard for diabetes control. Jennifer's glycemic control is mostly in the target range, and she has excellent glycohemoglobin levels. Her mother told us that during their visits with the pediatrician, he looks at the blood glucose charts and points out every high. Jennifer and her mother leave these visits feeling defeated, as though they can't do anything right.

We try to counter this approach. It is important for clinicians to have a positive, not negative, point of view. We believe strongly that people need to leave office visits with the strength to overcome obstacles. This doesn't mean that problems should be ignored. Rather, it is the function of the clinician to point out problems in a positive and constructive manner, without blame, and to suggest how the problems might be overcome.

One role of the clinician is to help children and their parents deal with their feelings. Allow them to feel angry, for example. But then try to shift the perspective. Help them to focus on their successes. It is necessary to point out the negatives when you think they are dangerous or risky, especially when you sense underlying risk-taking behavior. But it is just as important to notice and point out successes. Ask empathic, supportive questions such as "What's the hardest thing for you about living with diabetes, and how can we help you deal with that problem? What problems or behaviors do you want to work on now? What do you want me to work on with you? What would you like your goals to be?" Comments such as "You're eating THAT?" are not helpful.

Humor can be a tremendous help to lighten the load when things are getting too serious or discouraging. The psychologist on our team, who has written of his experiences with his son, Blake, who has diabetes, tells of Blake's struggle to add a second daily shot to his regimen. He and Blake got into a discussion of why a second shot was necessary, and the ramifications of fewer and fewer shots. Why not one shot a day? why not one a week? why not one a year? they asked, perhaps deteriorating into silliness. But after Blake and his dad laughed about how big a needle he would need for one shot a year, Blake had no problem with two shots a day.

SHIFTING RESPONSIBILITY

Diabetes is a family disease, and it affects the most basic components of family functioning—family routines, eating habits, planning, vacations, emergencies. The family must work together as a team for diabetes management. They soon learn that it isn't easy. Even in the DCCT intensively controlled group, only 5 percent of patients could maintain consistently normal glycohemoglobin levels throughout the duration of the study.

With the hormonal shifts and growth spurts and emotional issues of puberty, diabetes management can become even more difficult for teenagers. If teens and their parents are pushed to achieve glycemic control that is beyond their reach, this can lead to a sense of hopelessness. "I can't ever do anything right," the child will think, and this will lead to decreased motivation and contribute to even worse glycemic control. Medical goals must be realistic and fit the child's age and the family's abilities, but they cannot be set too low, because that would result in chronic hyperglycemia and long-term complications. It is necessary to set a middle ground—and to realize that this middle ground shifts throughout childhood, and particularly during puberty.

Gradually, the responsibility for diabetes care will shift to the child, but parental supervision should be part of the process every step of the way. Responsibility should not be shifted on the basis of age alone. Cognitive ability varies widely in children. If responsibility is transferred too soon, diabetes control is likely to worsen. When dealing with children in their teens, clinicians and parents must recognize that no one but the teen can control his blood glucose levels. It is not possible to force teenagers to do what they're not willing to do. Parents and clinicians can help, and they can and should work with the teen to support the goal that he has chosen.

Shifting responsibility can be very difficult for parents and health care providers alike, as Susan's case illustrates.

> **CASE STUDY.** Susan R. is a 10 year old who has had diabetes for 4 years. She has been accepting of her disease, and her glycemic control is generally very satisfactory, with glycohemoglobin levels of 7.2 to 7.9 percent (normal: 4.5 to 6.1%). When she turned 10, she and her parents felt that she was ready to take over full responsibility for giving her own insulin injections. Before that, she had been doing blood glucose monitoring successfully by herself and had mastered injection technique. She had been giving herself the injections for almost a year, after her parents drew up the insulin and as they watched. Now, she and her parents felt that she was ready to take over the responsibility for both drawing up and injecting. For 2 months, Mr. and Mrs. R. carefully observed Susan drawing up and injecting, and there were no apparent problems. They felt confident enough to stop watching.
>
> For several weeks, Susan's blood glucose level remained steady, but then it began to climb. Her parents noted high morning blood glucose and occasional morning ketones. They suggested that Susan increase her evening dose of NPH to try to correct the problem, but there was no improvement. When they questioned Susan in a gentle, supportive way about what might be occurring, she said, "I'm in too much of a rush at dinner to take my shot, and then I forget." Susan was not giving herself her evening injection on a regular basis. When her parents resumed close supervision, her blood glucose levels came back under control.

PROBLEM SOLVING

Diabetes management presents challenge after challenge to the problem-solving skills of clinicians, parents, and patients alike. It is important to include children in the problem-solving process as soon as they have sufficient cognitive skills to become involved.

The very specific problems of diabetes management must be attacked in steps, and all but the youngest children need to be aware of how one step leads to the next. Every principle can be illustrated with the very specific details of the child's diabetes management. During a clinic visit, it is helpful to start by identifying one area of living with diabetes which the child or teen wants to change. Ask the question, "What do you think you need to do to manage this problem?" This helps to crystallize the problem and paves the way for potential solutions. Emphasize that there is probably not one single answer for each question. Suppose that a child is eating a very large snack (about 800 calories) when she comes home from school, and her before-dinner blood glucose is soaring to 450 mg/dL. The possible solutions include eating a bigger lunch, so that her after-school hunger is not so great; eating a smaller snack; and covering the large snack with an extra dose of Regular or lispro insulin. The clinician can figure out the specific first step that seems most likely to address the problem. Signed contracts or written summaries of a clinic visit can often be helpful in reinforcing patients' and families' awareness of the problem-solving steps that need to be taken.

It might seem that covering every meal and snack with insulin is a solution to nearly all food-related problems and would allow the child to eat whatever and whenever she wants, but that is an oversimplification. First of all, this solution might lead to weight gain. Also, some children will complain that they don't want to have another shot, that they don't want to always carry their injection supplies with them, that they don't want to always have to calculate doses, and that they don't want to do the extra work involved with this level of management.

As the child or teen with diabetes grows up with all the medical and psychosocial strains added and aggravated by this disease, it is important for parents and clinicians to support the child's emotional strengths with trust, caring, and optimism. They must take care that diabetes management does not overcome the satisfaction of daily life or prevent families from enjoying and loving each other. This is sometimes easier said than done, and it requires awareness and work. Even the stresses of life without diabetes can sometimes be overwhelming for both children and adults. It requires that parents and children spend time together, talk openly, communicate honestly, and share their concerns and problems with each other and with the health care provider. And it requires seeking out psychological help when problems seem too difficult to handle alone, as the case of Cameron illustrates.

CASE STUDY.   Cameron H. was diagnosed with diabetes at 11 years of age, the first person with diabetes in his family. His father is a university professor and his mother is an accomplished artist. He has one older sister, and both of the children do very well in private schools. Cameron and his family learned the fundamentals of diabetes management and the skills of balancing a complicated regimen very quickly.

During the next 3 years, Cameron did very well. He told us that diabetes management (a three-shot-per-day regimen) was "easy" and that he didn't let it consume his life. Then, at age 14, entering adolescence, he became depressed, with flat affect and lack of enjoyment of life. He has a family history of clinical depression. Suddenly, Cameron began having a great deal of difficulty managing his regimen; his blood glucose levels were often out of the target range, and he had an elevated glycohemoglobin of 10.4 percent.

We referred Cameron for treatment for depression. At the same time, we simplified his regimen to two fixed shots a day and the same amount of food at the same times every day. Cameron's parents became more involved in his diabetes management. With his daily decision-making no longer so burdensome, and with psychotherapy and antidepressant medication, Cameron's diabetes management improved and his depression lessened.

The right attitude is important and can help. Diabetes control should be an integral part of the life of the child or teen with diabetes—but it can't take up his whole life. It needs to be an accepted element of daily life: it is something a child must do for himself; there is simply no choice about it. But it must be done in the context of a whole life. If a child is terrified of getting a long-term complication and devotes his whole life to preventing it, his life is restricted, just as it would be restricted if he were afraid of driving on the highway because of the fear of an accident and thus never drove on the highway. We can't ignore the fact that there are real risks for the person with diabetes, but a balance must be struck. Balance is the key.

PATIENT BURNOUT

It is not surprising that children and teenagers with diabetes will sometimes feel overwhelmed by the tasks of managing their disease. They may think that diabetes is taking over their life, that they are alone, and that no one else understands what they are experiencing. During these periods, many children will feel ambivalent about improved self-management—on the one hand, it may seem that this requires too much of a struggle for their efforts to be worthwhile; at the same time, however, they may feel guilty and fearful about the results of their poor self-control. This feeling of hopelessness, the sense that there is no solution, no way to alleviate what seems to be an unbearable situation, invariably leads to even less success in management.

It is during these times when patients are feeling despair that they have the greatest need for care and close attention from their health care providers. The clinician can heed the child's emotional needs and help her negotiate goals. This may be a critical time in the therapeutic alliance, and the provider should be aware of this. Sometimes the simple act of breaking down the tasks of diabetes control into small pieces and working with one piece at a time makes the oppressive duties seem more manageable to the patient. For example, for the child who is disorganized and hurried in the mornings and thinks that she just doesn't have time to take care of her injection, it can be helpful if a parent organizes all of her supplies in a little box, so that the entire burden is not on the child.

Most adolescents with diabetes go through a period of feeling that they can't cope. They think that their burden is too heavy, they let things drop, they stop being careful, and they stop monitoring. It is important that the clinician approach this with a supportive, not condemning, attitude. The clinician may be tempted to say something like, "Who do you think you're hurting? Not me, not your parents. You're hurting yourself." But such a strategy is likely to be counterproductive. Instead, the clinician could say, "You've really had a tough time these past 2 months. What are your feelings about this? What can we do to help?"

Don't underestimate the value of showing support. Sometimes we say to patients, especially small ones, "You really need a hug," and sometimes a hug can make a tremendous difference when people are going through difficult times. A good, empathic clinician will have a sense of when a hug is appropriate. It is best not to hug a child when a parent is not present. Sometimes a parent may need a hug, too, or a verbal equivalent of one.

CLINICIAN FATIGUE

Clinician fatigue or burnout results from a number of factors, all of which, unfortunately, are likely to increase in the current health care environment. Chief among these is high work-related stress, the feeling of being overworked and underappreciated. All too many clinicians today are experiencing a decrease in their satisfaction with their workload and sometimes with their interpersonal relationships.

Providing care to patients with major chronic diseases has its own set of frustrations and sense of futility for the clinician. This is often compounded by unrealistic goals and expectations on the part of patient and clinician, as well as the tendency of some health care providers to assume too much responsibility for problem solving.

If clinician fatigue contributes to less than optimal patient care, this deprives patients of their most significant ally. It disrupts the therapeutic alliance for the patient. The clinician needs to overcome these difficulties using all the resources at his or her disposal. The patient's family is the primary resource to help with treatment plans and goals. More personally, as a clinician you must strive for balance in your personal life. You can't take all the clinical burdens on yourself. Recognize that you don't succeed with everyone. Take a break. Talk to colleagues, family, and friends. Working with a team or with other providers can be helpful in preventing or detecting burnout. Working closely with a colleague can help you, and you can help each other.

IN SUMMARY, MANY ASPECTS OF LIFE WITH DIABETES can be burdensome for patients, their families, and clinicians. Conversely, though, there are strengths that can result from living with this disease and all the daily management tasks that are required. For instance, we see in some patients a healthy lifestyle with an increased awareness of the importance of physical activity and nutrition. Parents may feel that successfully dealing with all the day-to-day issues of diabetes care puts other aspects of life in a better perspective. Finally, children and teens with diabetes, and their families, may develop a deep sense of satisfaction and competence from their ability to live successfully with this disease.

12

Personal Perspectives of Children and Adolescents

This is a near-verbatim transcription of a lengthy conversation with the participants listed below. While they often referred to themselves as "diabetics," clinicians prefer to use the term "people with diabetes." In addition, their discussion of omitting insulin when ill is not correct sick day management (see chapter 8).

PARTICIPANTS

➤ Ellen—age 11
➤ Rachel—age 12
➤ Stephanie—age 12
➤ Mark—age 20
➤ Jack—age 16
➤ Jane (Jack's mother)—age 42
➤ Tom (Jack's father)—age 42

How old were you when you got diabetes, and what are your first memories of it?

ELLEN: I was 14 months old, so I don't remember much. Probably the first thing I remember was when I was at Camp Glyndon [a camp in Maryland for children with diabetes] and I tried to give myself my first shot without an injector. I was about 6 or 7.

RACHEL: I was almost 4 when I was diagnosed. I just remember drinking a lot and waking a lot in the middle of the night to go to the bathroom.

STEPHANIE: I was 11, and it was only 6 months ago. I was really thirsty, and I lost 10 pounds. I was thirsty for 3 days, and then I went to the doctor. My first thought when I found out I had diabetes was that I didn't want to give myself shots. I was scared of it. I knew because of my babysitter, she would do it right in front of me and I was like, how can you do that?

MARK: I was age 15, a freshman in high school. At first I was diagnosed as a borderline diabetic and I was just controlled with my diet, but I progressively got worse. The borderline phase only lasted about a month and a half. Then I started on the insulin shots. At first I couldn't give myself the shots, I was pretty much scared. Yeah, just taking your hand and piercing your skin. I would practice on an orange, but it just wasn't the same. I went for about 7 months without giving myself a shot. And then I started giving myself shots for around 5 months, and then I stopped for some reason. I don't know why.

But I finally went on a camping trip, and my parents weren't there. That forced me to give myself a shot. I really wanted to go on that camping trip because I wanted to be in a situation where I had to give myself the shots. So that's how I overcame that.

JACK: I was diagnosed at 9. The physical symptom I had was just a constant thirst. When I first got it, I was kind of upset, but not really. Because both my parents had it, so it had always been around my house. And it really wasn't that big of a deal. I mean it was kind of a big deal to take a shot. But I got used to it. It was just like something you've got to do. I'd seen my parents giving themselves shots all the time. I wasn't waiting for it to happen to me, it just happened, and I just took it as, you've got to do this or you'll get sick, you'll start feeling the way that you did before. That wasn't a good feeling.

JANE: It was a shock when Jack got it, even though Tom and I both have it, and there is a big probability that one or both of our children would have it. But when it comes, you're not ready for it. My father also had Type 1 diabetes, so I grew up with it, but I wasn't diagnosed until I was 21. I thought I'd escaped it; it was a little of a jolt.

TOM: I was 13 when I was diagnosed.

When you were diagnosed, did you feel you were different from the other kids?

TOM: I did. I was in a school population of about 1,600, and I think I was the only diabetic. This was in Dover, Delaware. And I dreaded the shots. For me that was the only thing about diabetes—I knew nothing of the disease, I just knew you had to take a shot. At that time I was on one a day, then eventually I took two. I was supposed to go to the doctor every 2 weeks to get a fasting blood sugar, and I might have gone every other month.

STEPHANIE: I just didn't want to tell anyone because I was afraid they'd feel sorry for me. It was like after they found out, they all became my best friend. They felt sorry for me and wanted to be my friend. They don't anymore, because they realize it's not a big thing, but before they were like, "Oh God, you have to give yourself shots, I feel so sorry for you."

How do you feel about giving yourself needles?

ELLEN: I don't really mind the needles that much. I don't think I ever really have, except for when I was 6 and the first time I gave myself my shots. Because I knew that I had to give it to myself, and if I didn't—I mean, I wanted to just get it over with, so I just did it. And if I didn't do it, my parents did. And since I've had it since I was 14 months old, that's just the way of life I know, so I don't really care that much about it, I guess you could say.

RACHEL: I'm going to Camp Glyndon this summer, and I'm hoping they'll help me, because I'm still really scared of giving myself needles. I practice on a doll, but I don't give it to myself yet. When I was first diagnosed they gave us this doll, and I colored on her and practiced on her. I put Band-Aids where I practiced giving her shots.

JACK: Giving yourself a needle started off hard at first, but once you over-come the little bit of fear you have with it, it's pretty easy. I wear an insulin pump now. I got it in April of last year.

MARK: How do you like the pump?

JACK: It's pretty good.

MARK: Do you feel high much anymore?

JACK: It keeps it pretty stable.

MARK: Do you play sports? [Jack doesn't.] I didn't get the pump because I was in sports. Playing soccer, basketball, just being that physical. I know you can take it off, but I don't mind giving myself the needles, so I didn't do it. But I'm having a little harder time controlling my sugar levels. I peak, get too high.

JANE [who also uses a pump]: I always would peak that way, too. Now it's more even. I have better control.

STEPHANIE: I don't like taking blood. It doesn't hurt that much because I have that medicine you put on, the EMLA [eutectic mixture of local anes-thetics] cream. But last week I had to get a gamma globulin shot in my hip, and my sister was just like, "Ow!" and I said, "Oh, that didn't hurt." It was a bigger needle, and I was scared at first.

Are there things about diabetes that you feel your parents don't understand? Your friends?

ELLEN: Not really. Maybe the fact that they don't really understand how it feels, but other than that, not really. My friends don't understand all that much, but they still help me a lot.

JACK: I think my parents understand pretty much, obviously. My friends— I mean, they know what's going on, but I don't think they know how it feels. You don't know how it feels unless you actually experience it.

RACHEL: I think my parents understand a lot what it feels like. Most of my friends have been in my classes since elementary school, and they basically know. If I feel low, they know what's happening. And they'll like take me to the nurse. I have to take a snack in school. Some people wonder why I have to take a snack, and others, they know. A lot of people understand why I have to eat in class, so I don't feel like I'm different. I sometimes don't feel like interrupting what I'm doing. I just take it out from my desk—I can be writing something and just every once in a while take a drink. What people don't understand is like when I'm at a party and everyone is eating M&M's, and I want to eat it, too. Sometimes I feel like saying, "I wish I could eat that, too." But it doesn't bother me that much. I mean, I basically understand.

STEPHANIE: My friends, they're always bugging me about what I'm eating, and I say, I've had my carbs, as many as I need. And my friends are always asking me if I can have what I'm eating. "Are you sure you can have that?" "Yes, it's okay."

MARK: You'll get that all the time, for the rest of your life, people watching what you eat. "Oh, you can't have that."

TOM: I've had a kidney-pancreas transplant. I don't have to take the shots anymore. The fortunate thing was, it's totally turned my life around. But unfortunately I lost my sight after the transplant. I'd had one episode before the transplant, where my sight really went bad. After the transplant there were a few episodes, and then quite suddenly it went altogether. And rather than it being retinopathy, which is a complication of diabetes and ruptured blood vessels in the eye, mine is a lack of blood flow to the optic nerve. Yes, it's diabetes-related, because any ischemic blood problem is always diabetes-connected.

How do you kids feel about Tom's blindness?

JACK: I don't know, it's kind of weird. It makes you think, is this going to happen to me? Is there any point in doing what I can to keep myself under control if it's going to happen anyway? Because there's a possibility that it could. But usually if you keep yourself under good control, it won't. But it kind of makes you realize that it's serious. A lot of people just blow it off with, "Oh, if I just take a shot, then I'll be all right." And it's not that; you've got to keep yourself under control a lot better. With my insulin pump, I can do what I want now.

ELLEN: I think it scares me a little. But it's like Jack said: I know that if I stay under control and if I try to keep my diabetes healthy, then I'm not as scared, but I'm still a little scared.

RACHEL: I really don't worry about that much. I haven't really thought about it. I just know if I stay healthy, and keep everything under control, hopefully, I'll be okay.

TOM: I know I was not well controlled as I was growing up. And to encourage the young people, you've got so much technology right now that I didn't have. I didn't have a doctor who was a diabetes specialist. I was diagnosed at 13, and I was 27 before I got a glucose meter. So I went through 14 years of who-knows-what before I even tried to get a handle on it. I lost my sight in May of '95, it's been almost 2 years. I'm totally blind, I see black. I had my kidney-pancreas transplant in October '93, and it works very well. I feel great, but unfortunately, I guess, the eyes and my toes were something waiting to happen. We didn't have any forewarning—it just reared its ugly head. I've lost all my toes because of poor blood flow. I didn't hurt them in any way to start a wound, but a wound created itself, and I've lost all 10 toes. I've had a transmetatarsal amputation of both feet. I've been given special inserts; I can wear sneakers or a boot or a shoe. And I make out very well. I feel that if I wasn't blind, I would have no trouble walking at all. I spent the first 18 years after high school training and driving harness horses. Now, since 1990, I've been an office manager at an insurance agency. I can still do that.

STEPHANIE: Having just been diagnosed, I think about things like complications because my doctor is always telling me. I'm not really good with my feet, I don't wear shoes and everything, and I'm always cutting my toes and things. And I'm worried I'm going to have bad circulation when I grow up and stuff. But I haven't had diabetes long enough to know everything that will happen to me. It's under control, but it's not as under control as I'd like it to be. But I'm hoping that after a while I'll get there.

Tom: I think control was an extremely big factor that I was able to ignore because I felt great. When I was 28 or 30, I felt indestructible. That's the part about diabetes that maybe fools you. But that's why I urge control. Because that's something you don't have any real handle on. I think I probably went through years of sugars in the 300s and 400s on a daily basis.

Mark: I worry about my eyes and my feet. Probably more my feet than my eyes. I know that occasionally, when my blood sugar goes high or low, my vision tends to get a little blurry or out of focus. I go every year to get my eyes checked, the whole nine yards, and they say I'm fine. My feet are iffy. I'm trying to strengthen the nails—I have really soft toenails and fingernails, and playing sports, they break a lot. And I get a lot of ingrown toenails. So I have problems as far as my feet. And I worry a lot.

Does having diabetes make you grow up faster or mature faster?

Mark: I would say that having diabetes makes you a lot more mature. Just as far as having self-control, saying to yourself, "I can't really eat that right now." Rachel is at a party, and she can't have those M&M's. We've all been there, and we all will be there again. You've gotta put the foot down—no, I can't have that. Each little bit makes you stronger and stronger.

Jack: I guess it makes me more mature, just because it's a lot of responsibility, keeping yourself under control. It's a lot of self-discipline, too. Like finally realizing, I have to give myself my shot. You have to discipline yourself to do what you have to do.

Are you kids being prepared better for life than other kids?

Jane: Yeah, I think so. I think that we're all thrown into growing up a lot quicker. You've got things to think about that most kids don't think of at all. Like, I have to take care of myself because I don't want to go blind or I don't want to lose my toes. And the responsibility of testing, taking your needles, making sure you have a bolus, you constantly have to think about it.

Do you ever feel you wish you could get a vacation from it? Do you ever wish you could have a day or a week without diabetes?

RACHEL: Sometimes I wish I could eat whatever I wanted to at any time. But other times, I normally eat what I would normally eat—I just don't have all this sugar. I can have some. When I was first diagnosed, I didn't eat that much sugar at all, and I ate a lot of things like sugar-free brownie mixes. But then the doctor said that I could start eating the regular brownie mixes. I eat more stuff now, and I decide what I eat by my blood test. Sometimes I wish I didn't have to do my blood tests or get shots every day. Sometimes I get bruises from the shots, and it hurts. Sometimes I wish I didn't have to do a shot until my arms would get better.

ELLEN: I think that a lot. And especially when I was younger and I used the injector. I did rotate my spots, but I always used the same general area, and because of the injector it caused big lumps. But they weren't bump bumps, like scaly lumps, they were just like my arms would come out a little bit from the injector. And that's when it was the worst ever, when I really wished I didn't have it. Now my lumps have gone and I don't use the injector so much anymore, and I haven't thought about it that much anymore.

JACK: A day or a week or the rest of my life. Yeah, you just feel like you need a break.

JANE: Tell them what happened when you took a break, when you went to the fair.

JACK: I had a severe low. I was about 10, the year after I got it. It was on my birthday; we were in Dover visiting my grandparents. The night before I had gotten low, and I had treated it. But I guess I didn't treat it as well as I should have, because we left real early the next morning. And I didn't test before we left. It was like an hour or something, I guess I passed out. They said I went into convulsions and all kinds of stuff. We were on the road, in the car. We ended up in the Elkton hospital.

JANE: We took a break, [and] figured, "Oh, it's your birthday, we'll check a little bit later since you got up earlier."

Jack: I don't really remember it. I don't remember actually being in the car. I just remember waking up in the hospital wondering what's going on. It scares you, if you come out of it looking at a whole bunch of doctor's faces. They told me right away that I'd gone low, and then they gave me a salad. And I was like, "Why are you giving me salad?" I said, "I don't feel like eating right now."

Have any of the rest of you had a bad low?

Jack: Oh my God, my mom passed out in her sleep. She had a seizure, it was a bad scene. We had glucagon, so I ran downstairs and got it out of the fridge, and then I was like, "Okay, I need to read the directions," and there were six pages of directions in little tiny print, you could barely read it. And I'm like, "Oh jeez." And the ambulance is on the way, and it was crazy.

Tom: I had insulin shock when I was about 17, after my junior class trip. I had taken a little extra insulin because I figured I'd cheat some that day. But I didn't take into account that we were going to walk Washington, D.C., from one end to the other. And the next morning my mom let me sleep in, and when I got up I remember coming out into the living room, and her giving me some eggs, and the next thing I knew I woke up in the emergency room. You don't remember it because you're passed out, and coming out of it you're so confused, you're still low. You don't have the strength hardly to react for a while.

Rachel: I was sleeping, it was a Saturday morning. My sister heard me making moaning noises in my room, and I was rolling over in my bed a lot. She got my parents, and they did my blood test, and I was low. My parents put sugar in my cheek, and they gave me glucagon and called the doctor. The glucagon made me throw up, and I got a headache.

Stephanie: I've had lots of lows. I haven't had a bad one yet.

Ellen: Well, I had one that wasn't serious at all. I mean, I didn't even faint. I was with my grandmother and my sister. I think we were coming back from the movies. I said, "Grandma, I feel low," and she said, "Ellen, just wait until we get home." Because she thought I was like joking or something. So we stopped to go to the bathroom because I really had to go, and I went into the stall and I shut it. And then I just sank to the floor. And since it was locked, my grandma couldn't get in the bathroom. She had to crawl under. And then she finally believed me. And then I think she had one of those little tiny tablets that's white and melts in your mouth.

JACK: BD tablets. They're like glucose tablets.

ELLEN: And she gave me one of those, and I felt better. But I didn't actually faint or anything. That was right before my grandmother really started to understand what was going on. I think I was really young when this happened—it was before I was even 6.

What does it feel like when you get low?

ELLEN: Well, a lot of times it's very hard for me to see, it gets blurry. And it's hard for me to walk, too—I feel very weak. And sometimes I feel like I might vomit, but I never really have, I just feel like it. And I feel like everything is spinning around me sometimes. And you get very confused, too.

JACK: Sometimes you get a shaky, nervous feeling, kind of. Sometimes I get in a real bad mood. I sweat. I'll get real hot, weak, tired.

MARK: When I get low, I'm sweaty. It's like when you see someone who has been drinking for a while, and they're drunk—their equilibrium is off and their balance is off. I have trouble walking; I walk on the wall pretty much. Some mornings I wake up and my arm will be dead, just have no feeling. Inside I get the butterfly-type feeling, that's the first thing. One morning I woke up—I work on cars a lot. And I was working on an engine. I was just excited. So I woke up, didn't eat anything, but I gave myself a shot. First mistake there. A friend was with me—he knew I was diabetic because I tell everyone. I figure the more people who know that I'm diabetic, the better chances I have of getting help if something happens. I was downstairs working on the motor, I was really having a hard time. I couldn't get anything to work, this bolt just wasn't going in, that wasn't working—like, forget it. My friends just thought I was upset because I couldn't get anything to work. I had overalls on. I took my overalls off and threw them into the corner. Next thing I remember I was eating ice cream. It's weird not knowing what you did for 4 hours. I had clothes on, next thing I know I'm sitting in the chair in boxer shorts. Woooo, it's a shock.

Tom: I think it's good that some of your friends know. Jane and I dated since we were kids. And I called her one morning on the phone, and I was talking very incoherently, was being mean. She said, "What's the matter?" and I said, "I don't like you anymore," and I hung up on her. She knew that wasn't me.

Jane: From my dad, I'd seen him get like that. We were on the beach one time, and he was walking like he was drunk, and all these people were looking at him. We quickly got him help. But I just knew something was wrong with Tom that time. So I went over on my bicycle and started feeding him right out of the sugar bowl.

Tom: She came to the door, and I was half-dressed and I threw my socks at her.

How do you feel about telling your friends?

Stephanie: At first I didn't want anyone to know, because I didn't want to be different from anyone else. I just told a couple of people, the ones who came to visit me in the hospital. But then everyone found out. And at my birthday party I had all sugar-free candy and they saw me testing myself, so they kind of figured it out. And then they told other people because they didn't know it was supposed to be secret. But then it was just like it didn't really matter anymore, so I just told everyone. I did feel a little ashamed at first, but not anymore. Now people ask me what my bracelet is, and I tell them.

Rachel: I don't mind people knowing that I have diabetes. When my friends sleep over, they see me getting my shots and getting my blood tested. Sometimes they see my mom drawing it. I don't care if other people know, because it will just help me. Like if I don't feel good in school, it will just help me—they'll tell the teacher. So it doesn't bother me.

Jack: I don't really care. Everyone that I know knows that I have it. Just from getting low while you're like hanging out with people. You're like, "I need to get a Coke, I need to get something with sugar in it." You tell them that, and they're like, "Why?" And then you just say, "I'm diabetic, I've got to get something." Then when they understand, like cool, they'll go get it for you.

MARK: That's the best part.

ELLEN: I don't care if people know. I don't think I ever have. But when I first went to school, I found it hard to tell people. So I told a couple of people who were my very close friends, and I was just like, "If anyone asks, you can tell them, I don't care." And that's basically how it started when I was little. Because I was very shy when I was little. But then I saw the way people reacted to it—like Jack said, they always got me stuff, and they did anything I wanted them to for a while, if I was like low or something. So then I was glad I had it for a while, actually.

Do you ever use having diabetes to manipulate things?

JACK: Aaaaah, I've been known to do that. If you're really bored in a class, really want to get out of it, you just go, "I need to go to the nurse, I don't feel well." And then you just go to the nurse and test your blood sugar. It doesn't bother me to test blood sugar, you test it, and if it's a little high, just tell her, "I'm just really tired," and they're like, "Okay, lie down in here for a while." You've got to use it for an advantage at least once in a while.

MARK: At least in high school, certain classes aren't very fun, so I'll think, hmmmm, I just had lunch, maybe I could pull it off. I didn't have that much to eat at lunch, I'll tell my teacher I have to eat some more and leave class. Or I almost went to the point of giving myself a little extra R [Regular insulin] so I could eat extra sweets, because I like sugar so much. I mix the two, I mix N [NPH insulin] and R. And I'd give 1 or 2 extra units of R —I knew I wouldn't fall dramatically. That was at first, when I was experimenting.

STEPHANIE: I haven't done anything like that. But a lot of my coaches, like my soccer coach, I'd tell her I was low, she'd yell at me, "You haven't had your snack, you're not supposed to get low in my class." Well, I'm sorry, but when you're exercising you can't help it. She's like, "You should have had more to eat." I was like, "I know what I'm supposed to eat." We'd have a soccer game and I'd forget to have my snack because I didn't know when it started, and she'd yell at me. And I'd say, "I'm sorry." So like a lot of my teachers understand it, but a lot of them don't.

JACK: I've had teachers like that before, and at one point I was low, I was getting kind of irritable. I was like, "I need to go to the nurse." And she's like, "No, you can't," yada yada. And I was like, "Well, I need to." And then she was like, "No, I think you just need to go sit down." And then I just left class and went to the nurse. Because I know if I need something. You've got to look out for yourself with this. If you just went back and sat down and then passed out or went into convulsions in the class, they'd feel really stupid. They'd feel really bad. It's just stupidity, ignorance.

STEPHANIE: I've gotten low taking tests in school. I was really worried—I got low taking a bio test that I didn't want to leave, because I was afraid my teacher wouldn't understand and was thinking I was using diabetes to get out of stuff. So I just sat there and I scribbled stuff down. And I actually did pretty well on it, I was excited. But I was really worried. I told her that I'd gotten low before she handed them back, so she wouldn't think I was just saying that in case I got a bad grade on it. But then I got a good grade, so it was okay, never mind. I also got low taking my exam. It's annoying. It's because when you're really stressed out, you get low a lot more easily. And I didn't bring food with me because I thought I'd have enough.

What do you worry about related to diabetes?

ELLEN: I worry about getting low and not being with anyone who knows about it. I worry about someday if, say, I'm at the mall and I'm with someone I'm not usually around, like a friend—but not a close friend—who doesn't know. And I go into a dressing room to change and I don't come back out, because I'm low and let's say I fainted. What will happen, because she may not know what might have happened. She may think I just went to get another size, and not go look for me. Or if I get stuck somewhere and I don't have my insulin with me. I don't always carry my insulin around with me, my mom sometimes does. But if I got separated from my mom and I got lost in the mall, and I was stuck there—I got scared of that once. A couple of times. Because I'd be there without any insulin or money to buy food if I got low.

MARK: I worry about my feet. And about traveling more than anything. Even going on a plane—the plane goes down, I'm the first person to die. You hate to think you made it through the crash, but died because of a low.

RACHEL: I worry about being stuck in an elevator without my insulin. Like being low, and I have my juice and crackers and I eat them, and then if I feel low again I wouldn't have anything. I'm afraid of getting low sometime when I'm someplace where I can't get food. I make sure I have plenty with me. When I go to the mall, I bring money with me. And if I'm with my friends we'll go, we can get something to eat there. Or if I'm just out, I normally take the little backpack with me, with juice and crackers in case I do get low.

JACK: Sometimes I'm worried that what happened to my dad is going to happen to me. I worry about—sometimes you don't know when you're going to get low, it's so unexpected. I drive now, and I'm worried, sometimes I'm afraid—like, say, I'm driving on a long, long trip, and I'm out in the country and there's no place to get a Coke and a candy bar.

Don't you always have something sweet with you?

JACK: Well, I'll do something stupid and forget to take something with me. And then I worry about that the whole time.

TOM: I found, as a kid or an adult, that if I had something on me, I wanted to eat it, not save it. And then I'd go and get low and be like, "Oh, I've got to go get something." It's a terrible temptation to have a candy bar or a roll of Life Savers around.

JANE: I hate Smarties, so I keep them around because I won't eat them unless I need them. That keeps down the temptation. We're all human.

TOM: There's nothing worse than having a Milky Way within arm's reach. The life expectancy of that Milky Way isn't very long around me.

MARK: Honey is the worst thing if you haven't had it in about 2 years. I was in art class one time, hard candy didn't affect me that much—it won't bring me back from a low or even make me high. So I had this candy, and it had a picture of a bee on it. I didn't really think about it—I was eating it, and the next thing I knew, this shot of honey went into my mouth, and I was instantly bouncing off the wall. It was total sugar shock. I never had so much energy in my life. I must have been in the upper 300s, definitely. It was the sweetest thing I ever had. It was just a little bit. I haven't had honey since then. It really shocked me, the taste and what it did.

STEPHANIE: I'm going to Vietnam in March because my dad was in the war and lived there for a while. And I'm going there for 3 weeks, and I'm really worried because I'm the pickiest eater you'll ever meet. Like I won't eat anything. I'll eat pasta, and I'll eat pizza, but I won't eat soups. The only soup I'll eat is Campbell's. For a while the only thing I would eat is chicken, and my dad says, "You're never going to survive." So we're going to have to bring peanut butter and jelly sandwiches all the way to Vietnam. I'm worried that I'm going to get low but I'm not going to want to eat anything there.

What has the effect of diabetes been on your being a picky eater?

STEPHANIE: Well, it hasn't really done anything because everything I eat is fine for diabetes. I eat pasta and hamburgers and lasagna and all that stuff, and I can still have all the stuff I had before, now. So it's not like a big change. It was a big diet change on how much I could eat and how long I had to wait for it. For a long time I'd be really hungry—I'd feel low, but it wasn't actually low, it was being really hungry. Because it wasn't how much I eat, but when I eat it. Normally I'd eat a little now and then a little later. Now everything I eat has to be in a meal, planned. So I was eating everything I normally eat, but at different times. So I'd get really hungry, but I'm used to it now.

JACK: Yeah, it does automatically have an effect. You're used to drinking Cokes and sugar sodas, drinking juice all the time. You've got to switch to diet. And it's definitely a different taste. You just can't go to a buffet—you can't just sit there and eat and eat until you're full. It's like, okay, I've had two pancakes and an egg, I think I'm done. But I do still go to buffets, I still eat whatever I want. I just cover it with the insulin. That's what's so good about the pump. If you overeat, you don't have to go, "Oh no, I forgot to take that extra 2 units I should have taken." The pump has a constant rate of insulin to keep you at a normal level all the time. So if you skip a meal or you don't have time to eat a meal, or if you skip a snack because you're not hungry, it'll keep you at a normal level.

Does diabetes affect your tastes?

RACHEL: I don't eat as much sugar. I like vegetables, and I eat healthy most of the time.

JACK: Not since I got the insulin pump. I pretty much eat anything I want. Yeah, I like sweets, but I'm not talking about that, I'm talking about quantities of food. I can absorb a lot more food now than I could before the pump.

MARK: I eat anything. I feel I can pretty much eat what I want.

STEPHANIE: I do like sweets. But some of my tastes have changed. I used to like Chinese food, but I don't anymore. And I didn't have candy for 3 weeks when I was in the hospital, and then after I got out I just got used to not having it. And some candies I don't like anymore. Candy seems a lot more sugary than it used to. I'll eat one thing of M&M's and think, I don't want to eat anymore, it's disgusting.

JANE: There was so much that we didn't understand when Tom and I were growing up, so much that the doctors didn't understand. We learned so much when Jack was diagnosed. How calories are important, how important testing is, what causes ketones when you get sick, why sugar affects other organs, that it was actually okay to have a cookie once in a while.

Do you feel like you deny yourself a lot of the time?

JACK: Before I had the pump I'd get hungry and eat anyway, and my sugar would be really high and no one would understand and I didn't want to tell on myself. With the pump, you can eat as much as you want and still cover it.

ELLEN: When I get home from school, it's the peak time I feel hungry usually. It depends how I feel. If I'm energetic, I'll eat and then go exercise, but if not, I'll eat something that fills me up but doesn't have a lot of calories, like a salad, and then go sit.

RACHEL: No, I don't feel like I deny myself. If I'm hungry after school, I'll have a pizza bagel.

STEPHANIE: I don't really feel like I deny myself. A lot of the time I don't feel hungry.

What's the worst thing that's ever happened to you because of diabetes?

JACK: I think dad knows the answer to this one.

MARK: Once I had diabetic ketoacidosis. I woke up, this was maybe about 2 years ago. I felt sick. I vomited and I felt that anything I had eaten, I would vomit. I ate breakfast and I vomited. So I thought, okay, I won't give myself a shot so I don't have to eat anything, so I won't get low. I was all by myself. So I just didn't take my insulin. Which was the worst thing. And I guess my blood sugar kept rising and rising and rising. I really felt lousy, and I didn't take my blood—I just didn't think of it. So I'm sitting there, didn't eat anything, next thing you know, I threw up again. I'm like, "Oh, man." The next hour, I throw up again. Man, what's going on? I actually timed it—every 15 minutes I threw up. Worst thing ever. After a couple more 15 minutes, my parents came home. They took me to the hospital because I kept throwing up. My blood sugar was really sky high. After I got to the hospital, I could just dry heave. Are you all grossed out?

JACK: It hurts.

MARK: I was sitting in the emergency room, I was actually lying on the table. I'm lying there, I couldn't breathe, it was the worst thing. When I took a breath, my chest hurt so bad, I don't know why. I threw up, and it was this green stuff.

STEPHANIE: I'm going to throw up just thinking about it.

JACK: I'm remembering my mom 2 weeks ago. She went through the same thing.

JANE: You feel so bad, you don't feel like testing blood sugar, you don't want to take a shot. You think, if you don't eat, you don't need insulin.

TOM: I had an episode when I was about Mark's age. I didn't have a glucometer, and I went through it for about 3 days, and I did not take my insulin because I thought, if you don't eat, you can't need any insulin. And I was wrong. My blood sugar was 650, and I was rushed to the hospital, hardly able to breathe because my blood gases were so out of whack. All the oxygen I was sucking in was not going to my blood.

MARK: They put in a stomach pump, a nice tube down my nose, it would really gross you out if I said what they brought out of my stomach. IVs, I had millions of IVs all over. But I don't remember anything after they put the tube down my nose. Next thing I realized, I'm going into the ICU.

TOM: When my sugar was 650, they gave me 50 units of Regular every hour. IV.

MARK: I never knew what my blood sugar was. I almost died.

Has diabetes ever kept you from doing anything?

ELLEN: I don't think it has stopped me from doing anything, but I think it's made things harder to do. Like sports. I've had to do a lot of things to play sports. Like drinking juice at halftime, eating a little something before and dinner after. That's the main thing that's been harder. And school has been a little harder than normal. All the things you have to do, like going to the nurse at lunch. I used to have to go to nurse, at lunch and before I went home. And that was a real big pain, and I messed up in class. It was a big nuisance to do. Now I just go some days at lunch and some days at the end of the day.

JACK: I don't think it's kept me from doing anything.

RACHEL: I don't think it's kept me from doing anything, except for not eating everything at parties and stuff.

STEPHANIE: Well, just basically school, because I'm missing a lot of my classes to go to the nurse's office. It was really annoying at first. I didn't bring my food to my class, and the nurse's office, that's where they keep all the sugar, and they have a box in the gym office. Now I carry stuff with me.

MARK: Actually, it has kept me from doing something. Philmont [Boy Scout camping reservation in the mountains of New Mexico]. Hiking. I tried backpacking in Boy Scouts, I used to do it before I got diabetes, but I just couldn't do it anymore. I always got low. I went on a hiking trip in the Appalachian mountains, this was getting ready to go to Philmont. I was walking, I stopped, I ate some sugar. Okay, we'll go. Hike up this hill. And we hiked up the hill. Hiked down the hill, hiked up the next hill. I need more sugar. I was just eating candy bars. So the rest of the group went ahead—it was just my dad and me. I would say that I couldn't hike. But other than that—and I could do hiking now, I have better control. Then I couldn't do it. I can do anything now.

Do you think that having diabetes has changed your personality in any way?

MARK: No. I am what I am.

JACK: Same here. It doesn't affect your personality. It might make you more responsible, but it doesn't change your personality. You're going to act with your friends the same way you did before. It's not like, well I'm diabetic, I'd better just sit down and be quiet. You don't feel excluded or out of anything. Well, you might if they're eating M&M's, but that's about it, and you can get over that.

ELLEN: I really wouldn't know, because ever since I remember my personality, I've had diabetes.

RACHEL: I don't think it's changed me. When I get low I tell my friends. It's like the same way when you have a headache, you tell your friends that you don't feel good. I don't think it's changed my personality.

JACK: It's not like it makes you worse in any way. If anything, you gain a little more responsibility, a little more respect from your parents.

STEPHANIE: I don't think it changes my personality. But you have to be more responsible, you have to be more controlling of what you eat, and everything. But I don't know how I act when I'm low or anything like that, so I'm not sure.

JANE: I think it just limits you in certain things. Like now that I'm older, I have a need for scheduling, but I don't think it really changes who I am.

Tom: We all share a disease, and it's an extra responsibility, but everybody has something to nag at them. Asthma is a terrible thing, or a parent with cancer, or a dysfunctional family. You can't become consumed by it.

How does diabetes affect your attitude toward life?

Stephanie: You're more careful about everything. Yes, it can be a burden. You have to act more grown-up, and you have to do what is healthy for you and not what you want to do. Like sometimes you want to go and eat whatever you want, or do some things that you can't. So you have to be more grown-up.

Jack: I agree with everything she said. It affects your attitude a little bit. You know that you've got to do what you've got to do to keep alive, to keep yourself healthy. But some days you'll feel you want to do something, you don't feel like fooling with it. And if you get that kind of attitude, that'll take you to bad habits.

Ellen: I think that it does change your attitude, but not by a lot. I don't think it changes your attitude toward your friends, or any attitude like that. But it changes your attitude towards— something like, when you get up in the morning, your attitude is, you have a normal life, but then again you don't. It's like you have two lives, but you do them both at one time. You have diabetes, and it is different, and you have a certain attitude toward that. I think I have a different attitude toward that than I do towards the rest of my life. Like, I have a bad attitude toward diabetes, but then my overall attitude toward life is good. So it's like you really don't change it overall, but you change it toward diabetes.

Rachel: I don't think it's changed my attitude toward life. I don't think I act differently with my diabetes than somebody else who doesn't have diabetes.

13

Research
The Path to the Future

Within a generation, there have been great advances in the technical aspects of diabetes care. The tight control that is possible today as a result of home blood glucose monitoring and glycohemoglobin measurements translates into fewer complications and healthier lives for many people with diabetes. The next generation can look to further treatment advances, and real hope for a cure and effective prevention. Children diagnosed today with diabetes can expect to benefit from a number of current investigations, some of which already have clinical applicability.

Research efforts can be classified into several categories:

> ➤ technical advances involving devices and insulin delivery methods;
> ➤ new forms of insulin;
> ➤ new hormonal treatments;
> ➤ prevention of complications;
> ➤ prevention of diabetes; and
> ➤ cure through transplantation.

DEVICES AND INSULIN DELIVERY

Numerous devices are under investigation to improve or simplify diabetes management. One of the most talked about is a noninvasive blood glucose meter. Such a meter has been promised for years—but unfortunately the reality is not yet on the horizon, with successful development at least several years away.

A noninvasive blood glucose monitor would read glucose levels through the skin using a wavelength of light such as infrared, without the necessity of a finger prick. The barriers preventing successful manufacture and use of a noninvasive meter have been threefold: lack of accuracy, lack of reproducibility, and expense. Children and their families and health care providers make important decisions based on blood glucose readings every day. Accuracy and precision are imperative. The devices that have been tested so far do not work for all patients, have a high percentage of inaccurate readings, and are also too expensive for practical home use.

Other sensor devices in development use low-level electrical current to remove tiny amounts of fluid through the skin, where some sort of glucose sensor keeps track of glucose levels with continuous readings. While this approach is minimally invasive, a potential concern is the risk of infection as the skin integrity is breached.

New methods of administering insulin have the promise to make insulin injections a thing of the past. Intranasal administration of insulin and inhalation of insulin through a novel aerosol spray device have been found to deliver the insulin effectively. Preliminary data in laboratory animals, in pigs, and in humans have been promising, but because of variability of the amount delivered and the effect, aerosol administration of insulin still has limited clinical applicability.

Several techniques are being investigated to deliver insulin transdermally. The low permeability of human skin has restricted this drug delivery method to compounds with low molecular weights, but a method using low-frequency ultrasound has been found to increase skin permeability. The key is to find a way for the insulin to penetrate in accurately reproducible amounts and with accurate timing, without compromising the integrity of the skin.

Another refinement is the implantable pump. Implantable pumps are already being used with some adult patients. These pumps still only pump insulin, and the wearer still must be the glucose sensor and computer. In an implantable pump, the reservoir is filled every few months at the physician's office. While these devices offer only some advantage over external pumps, they mark a stepping stone toward further advancement of pumps.

There is also the possibility of improving home management with glycohemoglobin home testing kits, which are currently in development. And data management systems with blood glucose meters offer continuing refinements with each new model on the market, with hookups to software programs that allow users to download meter readings into their home computers and plot the results on charts and graphs. These devices will continue to improve and to become accessible to increasing numbers of patients.

NEW FORMS OF INSULIN

With the addition of lispro, clinicians are already beginning to see the increased flexibility in regimens that "designer" insulins will offer. Molecular manipulation of insulin has the potential to broaden coverage options with customized approaches and to lead to even more closely regulated blood glucose levels. Researchers are now moving toward determining what other insulin effects are desirable, and what molecular changes are necessary to achieve such effects. This technical tinkering has the potential to lead to more uniformity in insulin duration and peak and the development of longer-acting insulins for smoother action.

OTHER HORMONAL THERAPIES

Clinical trials with a hormone called insulinlike growth factor I (IGF-I) are investigating whether this substance can be effective in lowering insulin doses and improving blood glucose control. Like insulin, IGF-I must be injected.

Amylin is another hormone that is produced by the beta cells, and researchers are investigating the possibility that it plays a role in glucose control. A chemical analogue of human amylin has been synthesized, and research is ongoing to determine whether taking synthetic amylin with insulin is more effective than taking insulin alone.

In addition, there are several new drugs available for the treatment of Type 2 diabetes. At some time in the future, some of these agents may be found to have a role in treating Type 1 diabetes:

> Acarbose (brand name: Precose) slows the absorption of glucose from the intestine.
> Metformin (brand name: Glucophage) decreases insulin resistance.
> Troglitazone (brand name: Rezulin) also increases the cell's sensitivity to insulin but is not effective without insulin.

Whether these drugs—all of which are effective when administered orally—will have an additional role in the treatment of Type 1 diabetes is unclear at this time.

PREVENTION OF COMPLICATIONS

Some new drugs show promise for preventing or delaying complications, and there are also a number of compounds in development or clinical trials which represent significant improvement in the treatment of complications. However, as has been emphasized throughout this book, good blood glucose control is the best way to prevent the complications of diabetes. Issues about blood glucose, blood pressure, and blood lipid control, as well as other risk factors (e.g., smoking) contributing to the development of complications, are discussed in detail in chapter 10.

Several new products offer other possibilities of prevention as well. Aminoguanidine (brand name: Pimagedine) decreases the formation of advanced glycosylation end products (AGEs). AGEs remain indefinitely in the body, accumulating in tissues, and appear to contribute to retinopathy, nephropathy, neuropathy, and blood vessel abnormalities. Clinical trials of aminoguanidine on adults with Type 1 diabetes and nephropathy are currently under way.

Aldose reductase inhibitors are another class of drugs under investigation. Aldose reductase, the first enzyme in the polyol pathway of glucose metabolism, causes an accumulation of sorbitol in a hyperglycemic state, which in turn contributes to the formation of cataracts, to diabetic neuropathy, and perhaps to other complications of diabetes. Inhibiting the action of aldose reductase could help to prevent cataracts and the development of nerve conduction velocity deficits. Laboratory studies are under way with aldose reductase inhibitors.

New treatments are also becoming available for impotence and wound healing, two of the chronic problems of many adults with diabetes. Nearly half of men with Type 1 diabetes experience some impotence by the time they reach their mid-40s. An injection of a vasodilator into the base of the penis has become a popular treatment. That technique is further refined with a procedure in which a tiny pellet containing the vasodilator alprostadil is inserted into the end of the penis via a single-use applicator rather than an injection, eliminating injection discomfort and possible side effects. A new oral medication, Viagra, is also effective.

Bioengineered human tissue (derived from the foreskins of circumcised babies) is being used to treat foot ulcers in patients with diabetes and is showing some promising results. The developers of one compound under investigation claim that it promotes wound healing and closure and provides a permanent replacement for the patient's destroyed dermal layer, and clinical trials are under way.

Finally, to prevent hypoglycemia, some new products are offered which contain uncooked cornstarch in combination with protein and sugar. The cornstarch provides a slow infusion of glucose from the gut. These snack bars may be useful as bedtime snacks to prevent overnight lows.

DIABETES PREVENTION

The larger work of preventing Type 1 diabetes itself is under study in the NIH's Diabetes Prevention Trial. The DPT-1 will test preventive therapies in susceptible first-degree relatives of people with Type 1 diabetes. The markers for susceptibility are positive islet cell antibodies, positive insulin autoantibodies, and a decreased first-phase insulin release during an intravenous glucose tolerance test. The theory is that administration of low levels of insulin before complete beta cell destruction has occurred will induce some immune modulation, perhaps producing immunologic tolerance to specific beta cell antigens, which will prevent further beta cell damage. The first phases of the trial, which is attempting to screen 80,000 first-degree relatives under the age of 45, will use subcutaneous insulin for high-risk individuals and oral insulin for moderate-risk individuals. Eventually, purified glutamic acid decarboxylase (or another antigen) may be used in another oral trial.

Another preventive therapy under study is the use of nicotinamide, a vitamin similar to niacin, which may have properties that prevent further beta cell damage in individuals at risk for Type 1 diabetes. A clinical trial with nicotinamide is under way in Europe.

CURE

Perhaps the most exciting possibility for children and teenagers with Type 1 diabetes is the prospect of a cure through transplantation. Two types of transplantation are under study: pancreas transplants and islet cell transplants.

CASE STUDY.   Tom C. is 42 years old and was diagnosed with diabetes at the age of 13. Tom is discussed here because he is a living example of the real possibility of a cure for diabetes. But his is also a cautionary tale, because he could also be offered as an example of most of the serious major complications of Type 1 diabetes.

For the first year after his diagnosis in 1969, Tom was on one shot of insulin daily. He took about 85 units a day of a mix of NPH and Regular, filling his U-80 syringe beyond the calibrated markings. After an episode of diabetic ketoacidosis when he was 15, Tom stepped up to a two-shot-a-day regimen. His adolescence was "normal," Tom says, but he hated injecting himself and had a "why me?" attitude about his illness, frequently feeling sorry for himself.

As an adult, Tom worked as a horse trainer, a job involving considerable physical activity. Because he frequently experienced lows in the evenings, he went back to one injection of insulin a day and seemed to be doing well. "I always felt invincible," Tom says of his health. "I always thought that as long as I felt healthy, nothing could be wrong. The trouble is, with diabetes, by the time you feel bad something is already very wrong."

During a routine ophthalmologic examination in 1983, Tom—not yet 30 years old—was diagnosed with diabetic retinopathy. His vision was not impaired, and laser treatments were successful in halting progression of the retinopathy. But the episode was a red flag. Tom started becoming more conscientious about blood glucose monitoring and learned that his control was difficult, with frequent—and often unexplainable—highs and lows. In 1987, he was turned down for life insurance because of proteinuria.

For the first time, Tom started to worry about his kidneys, although he had no apparent symptoms. His doctor emphasized good diabetes control, and Tom also began taking blood pressure medication. But his kidneys were inexorably declining. In mid-December 1991, he came down with what felt like a flu. After weeks of recurring and receding symptoms, he went to his doctor, who confirmed that what Tom thought was the flu was nephropathy, and that Tom had only 25 percent of normal kidney function remaining.

On a restricted low-protein diet, Tom felt better. His focus was on retaining the kidney function he still had, but he knew that he was on the road to dialysis. He began hemodialysis in January 1993, with three 3-hour sessions a week that Tom—younger by half than many of the other patients—hated. Three months later, he switched to peritoneal dialysis, which he could do at home. He could also infuse his insulin through the dialysis, and for the first time in 24 years he didn't have to take shots.

On the kidney transplant list since before he began dialysis, Tom had also decided to have a pancreas transplant. On October 6, 1993, he received the kidney and pancreas of a young man who had died of a head injury. His recovery was uneventful, and today, more than 4 years after the transplant, Tom has had no symptoms of rejection. He will continue to take antirejection drugs for the rest of his life.

His new pancreas has healthy beta cells that produce insulin, and Tom no longer needs exogenous insulin. But even though he no longer has diabetes, he continues to pay the price for years of erratic control. In January 1995 he noticed discoloration of his right big toe. By May, impaired blood flow necessitated amputation of this big toe. Within several months, the rest of the toes on that foot were amputated, and within a few more months his left foot was similarly affected. But Tom never saw his toeless feet. He had been experiencing some visual problems in the spring of 1995, but his loss of sight was abrupt. "May 6, 1995, was the last day I saw anything," Tom says simply. "Since then my world has been black." It was determined that his blindness was caused not by the usual form of diabetic retinopathy, in which blood vessels erupt within the eye, but by an ischemic condition that robbed the optic nerve of its blood supply.

No longer able to train horses, Tom works in his family's insurance office and is learning to cope with blindness. He compensates for the bilateral toe amputations with inserts in his shoes. And he is quick to inform people that even though his most serious problems came after his "cure" through transplantation, he does feel that he is cured of diabetes and that further deterioration of his health may have been prevented. "The only thing I have to worry about now is cancer from the immunosuppressive drugs," he says wryly, adding, "We're all going to die of something."

A growing body of evidence proves that whole and segmental pancreas transplantation works as a real cure for Type 1 diabetes. Many patients who have undergone these procedures go on to lead lives free of insulin injections. Most often these transplantations are done in combination with kidney transplantations in patients with end-stage renal disease.

There are three major barriers to widespread pancreas transplantation. The first is the scarcity of donor organs. This problem is somewhat mitigated for diabetes patients by the fact that a piece of the pancreas—about half the total mass—seems to provide the recipient with the needed function, while still leaving the donor enough of a pancreas for continuing healthy function. The possibility of living donors considerably improves the prospects for more extensive use of pancreas transplants. While pancreas transplantation remains relatively uncommon—about 7,000 such transplantations have been attempted worldwide since the procedure was first tried in 1966—it is an alternative for severely compromised patients.

The second problem is one that is faced with any organ transplantation—the problem of rejection. The powerful immunosuppressive drugs that are used to treat rejection often have serious side effects, including the risk of dangerous infections and malignancies. This is why organ transplantation is not usually done in otherwise healthy people with diabetes. However, newer generations of immunosuppressive drugs are promising safer prevention of organ rejection. The third problem is preventing diabetes from recurring in the transplanted pancreatic tissue. Currently, immunosuppressive therapy prevents this problem also.

Many see islet cell transplantation as the wave of the future, the best hope for a cure for people with Type 1 diabetes. However, the road to widespread implementation has been frustrating, and progress has been slow. In some patients, transplanted islet cells simply do not do the job—the recipients still need exogenous insulin. Success in others has fueled the continuing research, but difficult obstacles remain. The same problem with rejection encountered with organ transplantation persists, and patients with islet cell transplants still need continuous immunosuppressive drugs.

Encapsulating the transplanted islet cells may help to prevent rejection and guard against the recurrence of diabetes, but the technology to develop suitable biohybrid membranes remains elusive. Another problem is that the cells cannot be harvested from live donors, making availability a major issue. Xenotransplantation from animals—pigs seem to be a likely source—is a possible solution, and scientists are working to develop transgenic animals with genetically engineered islet cells that will not be rejected by the human body.

There have been tremendous research advances that have benefited people with diabetes, and the future is promising for additional scientific breakthroughs. Money for research, from both public (government) and private sources, is crucial to this effort. The American Diabetes Association and the Juvenile Diabetes Foundation are major supports. All of us who care about people with diabetes can contribute to this important effort.

Appendixes

Cost of Diabetes Supplies

Test strips (per 100)	$36–68
Meters	$30–100[1]
Lancing device	$14
Lancets (per 200)	$5–12
Syringes (per 100)	$12–20
Insulin (per vial)	$18

Note: Costs are approximate 1997 prices as advertised in *Diabetes Forecast*.
1. Trade-ins and rebates reduce these costs further.

Diabetes Monthly Record

Month/Year: _____

NPH a.m. [ ]

Sliding Scale-Regular/Lispro a.m.		
From	To	Dose

NPH p.m. [ ]

Sliding Scale-Regular/Lispro p.m.		
From	To	Dose

Day	INSULIN				URINE		BLOOD GLUCOSE						Comments
	a.m.		p.m.		Ketones	Time	Break-fast	Lunch	Dinner	Bed-time	Over Night		
	R* Dose	N** Dose	R* Dose	N** Dose									
1													
2													
3													
4													
5													
6													
7													
8													
9													
10													
11													
12													

* Regular/Lispro
** NPH

234

Day	INSULIN				URINE		BLOOD GLUCOSE					Comments
	a.m.		p.m.		Ketones	Time	Break-fast	Lunch	Dinner	Bed-time	Over Night	
	R* Dose	N** Dose	R* Dose	N** Dose								
13												
14												
15												
16												
17												
18												
19												
20												
21												
22												
23												
24												
25												
26												
27												
28												
29												
30												
31												

Diabetes Weekly Record for Insulin Pumps

	12M	1A	2A	3A	4A	5A	6A	7A	8A	9A	10A	11A	12N	1P	2P	3P	4P	5P	6P	7P	8P	9P	10P	11P
Monday																								
Carbs																								
Basal Rate																								
Bolus Insulin																								
Blood Glucose																								
Tuesday																								
Carbs																								
Basal Rate																								
Bolus Insulin																								
Blood Glucose																								
Wednesday																								
Carbs																								
Basal Rate																								
Bolus Insulin																								
Blood Glucose																								

Thursday

	Carbs	Basal Rate	Bolus Insulin	Blood Glucose

Friday

	Carbs	Basal Rate	Bolus Insulin	Blood Glucose

Saturday

	Carbs	Basal Rate	Bolus Insulin	Blood Glucose

Sunday

	Carbs	Basal Rate	Bolus Insulin	Blood Glucose

12M 1A 2A 3A 4A 5A 6A 7A 8A 9A 10A 11A 12N 1P 2P 3P 4P 5P 6P 7P 8P 9P 10P 11P

Pediatric Diabetes Clinic Assessment

Name:

Age: _____ Today's Date: _____ Completed by: _____

1. *Background Information*

   How long have you had diabetes? _____

   Is there a family history of diabetes? _____ Yes _____ No

   If yes, please list: _____

   Do you have other health problems? _____ Yes _____ No

   Describe: _____

   Hospitalizations:

Date	Reason	Place

2. *Insulin/Medications*

   What type of insulin do you use?

   _____ Human   _____ Brand Name

   _____ Pure Pork

   _____ Beef/Pork Mixture

   Please list time, type (NPH, Regular, etc.), and dose of insulin:

Time	Type	Dose

   Who draws up insulin? _____

   Who gives insulin injections? _____

   Sites used for injections:

   _____ Arms _____ Stomach _____ Other (please list)

   _____ Legs _____ Buttocks

   Have you noticed any changes in the skin where you give injections?

   _____ Yes _____ No If yes:

   _____ Sunken _____ Lumps _____ Other (list) _____

   Where do you store insulin? _____

238

Do you ever make changes in your insulin dose? _____ Yes _____ No

  If yes, describe: _____

Do you ever forget to give insulin? _____ Yes _____ No

  If yes, how often? _____

Medications other than insulin:

Name of Medication   *Reason for taking*

_____   _____

_____   _____

Allergies? _____ Yes _____ No

  List: _____

3. *Monitoring*

Do you do _____ Blood _____ Urine glucose monitoring?

Type of equipment _____

Frequency and timing of tests _____

What are the usual blood sugar results for a typical day?

_____ Before Breakfast _____ Before Dinner _____ Other

_____ Before Lunch _____ Before Bedtime Snack

What range would you like to see your blood sugars? _____ to _____

At what blood sugar levels do you make changes in your care? _____

  Describe changes: _____

Do you test urine for ketones? _____ Yes _____ No

  When? _____

What type of testing equipment? _____

Do you keep a record of blood sugar and ketone results? _____ Yes _____ No

4. *Hypoglycemia*

How often do you have insulin reactions? _____ per month

Please describe how you feel and what you do to treat an insulin reaction.

_____

_____

If you have had any severe reactions, describe: _____

_____

What time of day do reactions occur? _____

What, if any, sugar source do you carry with you to treat reactions?

_____

Have you ever used glucagon? _____ Yes _____ No

Do you have glucagon in your house? _____ Yes _____ No

Does a family member know how to use it? _____ Yes _____ No

5. *Hyperglycemia/Ketoacidosis*

    Is there a recent history of getting up at night to use the bathroom or bedwetting?

    _____ Yes _____ No

    If yes, how often? _____

    What effect, if any, does stress have on your blood sugar? _____

    Have there been any episodes of ketoacidosis (diabetic coma)?

    _____ Yes _____ No   If yes, describe: _____

6. *Diet*

    Do you take vitamins and/or minerals? _____ Yes _____ No

    If yes, what kind? _____

    Food Likes   *Food Dislikes*

    _____   _____

    _____   _____

    _____   _____

    _____   _____

    _____   _____

    When was the last time your diet was reviewed by a dietitian? _____

    How many calories are you allowed on your present diet? _____

    How would you rate how well you follow your diet?   _____ Good _____ Fair _____ Poor

    Who does the food shopping? _____ Cooking? _____

    Do you have any financial difficulties with the food budget? _____ Yes _____ No

    Do you have any special concerns about the diet? _____ Yes _____ No

    If yes, describe: _____

7. *Exercise*

    Do you have a regular (at least 3 times per week) exercise program?

    _____ Yes _____ No   If yes, describe: _____

    What type of exercise do you enjoy? _____

    Do you make changes in your meal plan or insulin based on exercise?

    _____ Yes _____ No   If yes, describe: _____

8. *Education*

    Where did you have initial diabetes education? _____

    When was the last time you had a review of diabetes? _____

    Are you a member of   ____ ADA ____ JDF

    Have you attended camp? _____ Yes _____ No

    List any areas where you would like more instruction. _____

    _____

9. *Lifestyle and Daily Routine*

    Name of School: _____

Grade: _____

Name of School Nurse: _____

Phone Number of School: _____

How many days of school per year are missed because of diabetes-related problems? _____

    because of other problems? _____

Average Grades _____

Schedule (indicate time):

_____ School starts _____ Lunch _____ Gym (recess) _____ Ends

What snacks and sugar source do you keep at school? _____

Where at school is this kept? _____

Are school personnel helpful? _____ Yes _____ No

    Describe: _____

Do you receive any special education? _____

List any afterschool activities or job: _____

Are there any special weekend activities that change diabetes management (i.e., job, sports,

    more or less active)? _____ Yes _____ No

    If yes, describe: _____

Do you wear a Medic Alert bracelet or necklace? _____ Yes _____ No

Do you receive reimbursement for supplies? _____ Yes _____ No

Do you have difficulty paying for supplies? _____ Yes _____ No

What are parents' most significant concerns relating to diabetes on a daily or

    long-term basis? _____

_____

How do you feel about having diabetes? _____

_____

_____

What one thing bothers you the most about diabetes? _____

_____

_____

Are friends and family members helpful regarding diabetes management?

_____ Yes _____ No   Describe: _____

_____

Who lives in household? _____

_____

Please list family members who are involved in diabetes care. _____

_____

What do they do? _____

_____

_____

Please identify any other special concerns. Also, list anything else you want us to know about you and your family. _____

_____

_____

_____

_____

Thank you for completing this assessment.

Diabetes Patient Education Record

Patient Name: _____ History Number: _____ Date of Birth: _____

KEY CODE

Method:	**Participants:**	**Evaluation:**
A = audiovisual;	C = child;	D = demonstration of skills;
E = explain;	M = mother;	V = verbalizes understanding;
D = demonstrate;	F = father;	W = written knowledge.
P = printed material.	S/O = significant other.	

Date	Content	Method	Participants	Instructor	Evaluation
	1. *General Facts:*				
	Definition				
	Pathophysiology				
	Metabolism of CHO, protein, fat				
	Classification				
	Honeymoon				
	Treatment				
	Research				
	2. *Psychological Adjustment:*				
	Living with a chronic illness				
	Coping with daily demands				
	Availability of counsel and social worker				
	3. *Family Involvement:*				
	Diabetes as a family challenge				
	Support groups				
	Information for school personnel				
	Sharing responsibilities				
	4. *Nutrition:*				
	Individualized meal plan				
	Composition of meal plan				
	Resources				
	Achieving and maintaining body weight				
	Appropriate growth and development				
	Relationship to glucose control				
	5. *Exercise:*				
	Benefits				

Date	Content	Method	Participants	Instructor	Evaluation
	Exercise: Types				
	Precautions				
	Food and insulin adjustment				
	6. *Medications:*				
	Insulin				
	Source				
	Brand				
	Type				
	Action				
	Storage				
	Expiration				
	Drawing up				
	Mixing				
	Injection technique				
	Sites				
	Rotation				
	Syringes				
	Special Precautions:				
	Leakage				
	Lipohypertrophy				
	Lipodystrophy				
	Absorption rates				
	Injection times				
	Multiple injections				
	Insulin pump				
	Insulin pen				
	Injection aides				
	7. *Relationship between Nutrition, Exercise, Medication*				
	Adjustment of one factor in relation to another				
	8. *Monitoring:*				
	Goals				
	Types of monitoring				
	Interpreting blood glucose results				
	Finger sticking				

Date	Content	Method	Participants	Instructor	Evaluation
	Frequency of monitoring				
	Recordkeeping				
	Maintenance and quality control of meters				
	HbA$_{1C}$				
	Urine ketones				
	Lab work				
	9. *Hypoglycemia/Hyperglycemia:*				
	Definition				
	Signs/symptoms				
	Causes				
	Prevention				
	Treatment				
	When to call health care team				
	Glucagon				
	10. *Illness:*				
	Sick day management				
	Monitoring of blood glucose/ketones				
	Insulin dose adjustment				
	When to call health care team				
	11. *Complications:*				
	Acute				
	Hypoglycemia				
	DKA				
	Intermediate				
	Growth/Weight				
	Pregnancy				
	Long-term				
	Eye				
	Kidney				
	Nerve				
	Circulatory				
	Foot				
	Possible causes				
	Preventions				
	Monitoring				
	Treatment				

Date	Content	Method	Participants	Instructor	Evaluation
	12. *Hygiene/Health Habits:*				
	Yearly ophthalmology exam				
	Routine dental care				
	Smoking				
	Alcohol				
	Birth control				
	Drugs				
	Driving a car				
	Travel guidelines				
	13. *Benefits and Responsibilities of Care:*				
	Rights of patient				
	Responsibility of patient and family				
	Responsibility of health care team				
	14. *Use of Health Care System:*				
	Follow-up visits				
	Telephone calls				
	Emergencies				
	Specialty care				
	Financial assistance				
	15. *Community Resources:*				
	ADA				
	AADE				
	JDF				
	Diabetes camp				
	Special community programs				
	Literature				

Letter to Teachers of a Child with Diabetes from the Parent

Dear _____ ,

My child, _____ , has diabetes and takes insulin but should be treated as much as possible like any other child in the classroom.

Before lunch, or after exercise, or during stress, my child might have an insulin reaction (hypoglycemia, or low blood sugar). This reaction can come on suddenly.

Signs of an insulin reaction are: excessive sweating, faintness, pallor, headache, pounding of heart, trembling, impaired vision. Also irritability, crying, confusion, poor coordination, inability to concentrate, nausea, hunger, or inappropriate behavior. Although my child has been told to look out for these signs, my youngster may not recognize that a reaction is occurring. The reactions sometimes may be quite severe.

If you see these signs, immediate action is required. If you are in doubt, please go ahead with the following actions, and assess the situation later:

—Give my child some glucose (sugar) immediately, from the kit I have provided, or any of the following alternatives (you may need to do some coaxing):

glucose gel or tablets (follow instructions on the label);

2 large sugar cubes or 3 teaspoons sugar in a small glass of water;

½ cup fruit juice;

½ cup soda pop (containing sugar, not diet or sugar-free);

candy, such as 10 gumdrops or 6 jelly beans.

If my child is unconscious or unable to swallow, get emergency help.

—Do not leave my child alone. Get someone to contact me and my child's doctor at once. My child should improve within 10 minutes; if not, treat again. After an insulin reaction, my child needs additional food to prevent a recurrence of the reaction. Milk or cheese and crackers are good food choices.

There may be non-emergency situations, too. If there's a long time before the scheduled meal, my child may need some long-acting carbohydrate, such as graham crackers or _____ . Once my child eats this food booster, activities need not be restricted.

I am _____ (your name), and I can be contacted at _____ . My child's doctor is Dr._____ , and can be reached at:

Adapted from a booklet published by the Montana affiliate of the American Diabetes Association, *Clinical Diabetes,* September/October 1984, 117.
Courtesy American Diabetes Association

Letter to Teachers of a Child with Diabetes from the Physician

Dear (Teacher):

_____ has Type 1 insulin-dependent diabetes mellitus. This does not interfere with any normal activity, including physical education or gym. However, it may be necessary for him/her to have an extra snack before or after rigorous exercise. It may also be necessary to have snacks at school on a regular basis, in order to balance insulin intake and to try to maintain a close-to-normal blood glucose level. Teachers and all school personnel should be aware of the signs and symptoms of hypoglycemia (*low* blood sugar). These may include:

1. dizziness
2. shakiness
3. sweatiness
4. sleepiness
5. headaches

6. confusion
7. pale appearance
8. change in personality, such as inappropriate crying or laughing or inability to concentrate

When these signs occur, treatment is needed *immediately* or the problem will worsen. The treatment is to give food or drink containing sugar. Fruit juice, soda (not diet), sugar or honey may all be used. Parents may also provide you with commercially prepared items such as BD glucose tablets, Glutose, Insta-glucose, or Cake Mate icing. If symptoms do not subside in 10 minutes, repeat treatment. If a meal or snack is not scheduled within 15 minutes, follow the treatment with a snack such as milk or cheese. We advise students to carry sugar with them to treat episodes of hypoglycemia. Severe low blood sugar can result in loss of consciousness or seizures. This is a rare occurrence but requires treatment with glucagon (a prescription medication by injection) given by the nurse—or call 911 for assistance.

Signs and symptoms of too *high* glucose include:

1. excessive and frequent urination
2. excessive thirst
3. sleepiness

Notify parents if these symptoms occur.

If you have any questions or concerns regarding _____ ,
please call _____ .

Sincerely,

Problem List and Critical Pathway, New-Onset Diabetes after DKA

Primary Nurse _____

M.D. _____

Case Manager: _____ DRG – 295

Date to begin: _____ ICD9–250.1, 250

Date Initiated	Problem List (R/T) related to	Date Discussed w/ Pat/Fam	Outcome	Date Resolved
	1. New onset diabetes.		By discharge, patient will have stable blood glucose (80–200) and negative urine ketones. Patient will be tolerating ADA diet. Patient's SQ insulin dose determined.	
	2. Lack of knowledge about discharge and follow–up needs.		By discharge patient will be able to state: 1. date, time, place of follow–up 2. Meds: dose, route, schedule, side effects 3. diet and activity 4. reportable signs or symptoms 5. MD and RN contact number	
	3. Dehydration		At discharge, patient will be adequately hydrated as evidenced by: 1. equal I&O 2. tolerating po fluids/diet 3. stable Vs	
	4. Lack of knowledge about diabetes self care.		By discharge, patient/family will be able to state/demonstrate the content presented in the Diabetes Teaching Plan. *See Teaching/Learning Flowsheet	

Critical Pathway

Date: _____
Date discussed with patient/family: _____
Primary Nurse: _____
Attending: _____
Case Manager: _____

	Day 1 (Begins with conversion to SQ insulin)	Day 2	Day 3 Day of Discharge		
ASSESSMENT/ MONITORING	Blood glucose levels: before meals, bedtime, snacks (if needed) and between 2 and 3 am Urine testing for Ketones qd or BID if sick or Blood glucose ▲ 300 Strict I+O Vital signs q shift Nutrition Assessment called (Call Nutrition consult on admission: Ext 5 - 5177 or page 232 - 1024) Social Work Assessment initiated	Social Work Assessment completed Child Life Assessment			
TREAT-MENTS		Social Work counseling	Social Work inpatient counseling completed		
LINES/ DRAINS	IVF ➤ KVO or HL as per individual patient need	D/C IV if eating well			
MEDICATIONS	Convert to SQ insulin: (use Harriet Lane as a guide) • before meals • dose as per individual patient needs • regular insulin before breakfast and lunch or may begin NPH and regular pre-breakfast and pre-dinner • supplement with regular insulin pre-lunch and bedtime BG ▲ 300	Adjust insulin based on blood glucose levels	Discharge patient with insulin dose and contact numbers for follow-up and problem solving		

	Day 1	Day 2	Day 3
ACTIVITY	As desired and tolerated --------- OOB walking -------- Diversional activities	Medical play (when age appropriate) --------	
DIET	Begin ADA diet with snacks as prescribed --------		
TESTS			Anytime after DKA resolves and prior to discharge. Can be done inpatient or as outpatient. Hemoglobin A1C Fasting lipids Chemistry panel Thyroid antibodies TSH
PATIENT TEACHING	1. Family version of path shared 2. Standard Teaching plan for orientation to unit initiated 3. Teaching Initiated per Diabetic Standard Teaching plan Lesson I: 　Pathophys of diabetes 　Psychomotor skills 　Begin nutrition Instruction	Lesson II: 　Insulin and Insulin adm 　Nutrition 　Hypo/Hyperglycemia 　Blood glucose monitoring 　Honeymoon period	Lesson III: 　Review I and II 　General health measures: sick day & glucagon
DISCHARGE PLANNING	Prescription signed and given to family for: 1. Syringes 2. One Touch II Blood Glucose Meter and starter supplies 3. One Touch Blood Glucose strips 4. Lancets for blood glucose monitoring 5. Urine ketone strips 6. Glucagon Emergency Kit 7. Instant glucose 8. Regular and NPH insulin NOTE: Prescriptions are to be given to family on admission. Request they fill them ASAP.	Filled prescriptions presented to RN -------- Family used One Touch II (or home monitor) -------- Referral to home care made --------	At least one parent/family member has given insulin before discharge. Child's school contacted re: 　Medical & Nursing plan of care.

251

Critical Pathway, *continued*

Name: _____ Date: _____

EVALUATION OF OUTCOMES			
Assessment/Monitoring	• Blood glucose < 300 □ yes □ no • Negative Urine Ketones □ yes □ no • Nutrition Assessment initiated □ yes □ no Social Work Assessment initiated □ yes □ no	• Blood glucose < 300 □ yes □ no • Negative Urine Ketones □ yes □ no • Nutrition Instruction begun □ yes □ no Social Work Assessment completed □ yes □ no Child Life Assessment Completed □ yes □ no	• Blood glucose = 80 - 200 □ yes □ no • Negative Urine Ketones □ yes □ no • Nutrition Instruction completed □ yes □ no Social Work Inpatient Counseling completed □ yes □ no
Drains	• IV fluids to KVO □ yes □ no	• IV D/C or HL □ yes □ no	• Patient tolerating po fluids □ yes □ no
Meds	• Regular insulin before breakfast □ yes □ no • lunch □ yes □ no or NPH and regular insulin pre-breakfast and dinner □ yes □ no • Supplemental regular insulin needed before lunch □ yes □ no • before bedtime □ yes □ no	• Insulin dosage adjusted as needed □ yes □ no	• D/C dose of insulin determined □ yes □ no
Activity	OOB □ yes □ no	OOB □ yes □ no Medical play (when age appropriate) □ yes □ no □ N/A	OOB □ yes □ no
Diet	• ADA diet initiated □ yes □ no	• ADA diet tolerated □ yes □ no	• ADA diet tolerated □ yes □ no
Education	• Diabetic Instruction - Lesson I Completed □ yes □ no • Patient/Family verbalize understanding □ yes □ no	• Diabetic Instruction - Lesson II Completed □ yes □ no • Patient/Family verbalize understanding □ yes □ no	• Diabetic Instruction - Lesson III Completed □ yes □ no • Patient/Family verbalize understanding □ yes □ no
D/C	• Prescriptions given to family □ yes □ no	• Prescriptions filled □ yes □ no • Home Care Referral made □ yes □ no	• Family/Pt used/touch machine □ yes □ no • Family member administered insulin prior to discharge □ yes □ no • Patient/Family verbalizes understanding of D/C instructions □ yes □ no School contacted □ yes □ no
Tests			Done prior to D/C: Hbg A1C Fasting Lipids Chemistry panel Thyroid Antibodies TSH If not done inpatient, tests are scheduled to be done at outpatient visit **Pt. discharged yes no** □ yes □ no
Night	P A	P A	P A
Day			
Evening			
Signature/Title			

New-Onset Diabetes (after DKA) Problem List and Critical Pathway

Resources

THE AMERICAN DIABETES ASSOCIATION AND THE JUVENILE DIABETES FOUNDATION

All clinicians caring for children and adolescents with diabetes should join the American Diabetes Association and the Juvenile Diabetes Foundation and receive their publications. The ADA's *Diabetes Forecast* and the JDF's *Countdown* are excellent sources of patient- and family-oriented information. In addition, the ADA publishes many valuable books for professionals and families. Every year, *Diabetes Forecast* publishes a *Buyers Guide* that offers a detailed comparison of all diabetes supplies. To purchase ADA books, call 1-800-ADA-ORDER (1-800-232-6733).

The *Diabetes Resource Catalog* lists ADA publications that offer a wealth of information. A review of this catalog will help you to identify books that meet your specific needs. For a sampling of ADA books, see the ADA publications listed under "Recommended Readings," below. The American Association of Diabetes Educators (AADE) also offers valuable publications, including the *Diabetes Educator*, and provides a list of certified diabetes educators.

RECOMMENDED READINGS

Anderson, B., and R. Rubin, eds. *Practical Psychology for Diabetes Clinicians.* Alexandria, Va.: American Diabetes Association, 1996.

Becker, D. "Complications of Insulin-Dependent Diabetes Mellitus in Childhood and Adolescence." In *Pediatric Endocrinology*, 3d ed., edited by F. Lifshitz, 583–605. New York: Marcel Dekker, 1996.

Betschart, J. *It's Time to Learn about Diabetes* (workbook and video). Minneapolis, Minn.: Chronimed, 1991.

Betschart, J., and S. Thom. *In Control: A Guide for Teens with Diabetes.* Minneapolis, Minn.: Chronimed, 1995.

Brackenridge, B., and R. Rubin. *Sweet Kids.* Alexandria, Va.: American Diabetes Association, 1996.

Chase, P. *Understanding Insulin-Dependent Diabetes Mellitus,* 8th ed. Denver, 1995.

> Known as the "Pink Panther" book, this is an excellent and detailed guide for families. We believe that beginning at the time of diagnosis, all families should own either this book or *An Instructional Aid on Insulin-Dependent Diabetes Mellitus,* by L. Travis (listed below).

Diabetes Control and Complications Trial Research Group. "The Effect of Intensive Treatment of Diabetes on the Development and Progression of Long

Term Complications in Insulin Dependent Diabetes Mellitus." *New England Journal of Medicine* 329:977, 1993.

Diabetes Education Goals. Alexandria, Va.: American Diabetes Association, 1995.

Drash, A. *Clinical Care of the Diabetic Child*. Chicago: Year Book, 1987.

———. "Diabetes Mellitus in the Child: Classification, Diagnosis, Epidemiology, and Etiology." In *Pediatric Endocrinology*, 3d ed., edited by F. Lifshitz, 555–65. New York: Marcel Dekker, 1996.

———. "Management of the Child with Diabetes Mellitus: Clinical Course, Therapeutic Strategies, and Monitoring Techniques." In *Pediatric Endocrinology*, 3d ed., edited by F. Lifshitz, 617–29. New York: Marcel Dekker, 1996.

Farkas-Hirsch, R., ed. *Intensive Diabetes Management*. Alexandria, Va.: American Diabetes Association, 1995.

Frederickson, L., ed. *The Insulin Pump Therapy Book: Insights from the Experts*. Sylmar, Calif.: MiniMed, 1995.

Lawlor, M., L. Laffel, B. Anderson, and A. Bertorelli. *Caring for Young Children with Diabetes: Professional Manual*. Boston: Joslin Diabetes Center, 1996.

———. *Caring for Young Children with Diabetes: Parent Manual*. Boston: Joslin Diabetes Center, 1996.

MacCracken, J. *The Sun, the Rain, and the Insulin: Growing Up with Diabetes*. Orono, Maine: Tiffin Press, 1996.

Mazur, M., P. Banks, and A. Keegan. *The Dinosaur Tamer and Other Stories for Children with Diabetes*. Alexandria, Va.: American Diabetes Association, 1995.

Plotnick, L. "Insulin-Dependent Diabetes Mellitus." *Pediatrics in Review* 15:137–48, 1994.

"Report of the Expert Committee on the Diagnosis and Classification of Diabetes Mellitus." *Diabetes Care*, suppl. 1, 21:S5–19, 1998.

Rubin, R., J. Bierman, and J. Toohey. *Psyching Out Diabetes: A Positive Approach to Your Negative Emotions*. Los Angeles: Lowell House, 1992.

Santiago, J., ed. *Medical Management of Insulin-Dependent (Type 1) Diabetes*, 2d ed. Alexandria, Va.: American Diabetes Association, 1994.

Saudek, C., R. Rubin, and C. Shump. *The Johns Hopkins Guide to Diabetes for Today and Tomorrow*. Baltimore: Johns Hopkins University Press, 1997.

Siminerio, L., and J. Betschart. *Raising a Child with Diabetes*. Alexandria, Va.: American Diabetes Association, 1995.

"Standards of Medical Care for Patients with Diabetes Mellitus." *Diabetes Care*, suppl. 1, 21:S23–S31, 1998.

Travis, L. *An Instructional Aid on Insulin-Dependent Diabetes Mellitus*, 11th ed. Austin, Tex., 1996.

> This is an excellent and detailed guide for families. We believe that beginning at the time of diagnosis, all families should own either this book or *Understanding Insulin-Dependent Diabetes Mellitus*, by P. Chase (listed above).

White, N. "Diabetes Mellitus in Children." In *Rudolph's Pediatrics*, edited by A. Rudolph, 20th ed., 1803–27. Stanford, Conn.: Appleton and Lange, 1996.

Wysocki, T. *The Ten Keys to Helping Your Child Grow Up with Diabetes.* Alexandria, Va.: American Diabetes Association, 1997.

WEBSITES FOR PEOPLE WITH INTERNET ACCESS

American Association of Diabetes Educators: http://www.aadenet.org.
American Diabetes Association: http://www.diabetes.org.
American Diabetes Association, *Diabetes Forecast* magazine: http://www.diabetes. org/DiabetesForecast.
American Diabetes Association Publications: http://www.ada.judds.com.

A listing of books, journals articles, and the like.

CenterWatch Clinical Trials Listing Service: http://www.centerwatch.com.
"Children with Diabetes" homepage: http://www.castleweb.com/diabetes.

This site has specific information about and for children and teenagers. Some information is provided from medical sources and some from lay sources. "On-Line Links" helps you connect to other diabetes sources.

Diabetes Interview newspaper homepage: http://www.diabetesworld.com.
Juvenile Diabetes Foundation (JDF): http://www.jdfcure.com.
National Institutes of Health, Centers for Disease Control and Prevention: http://www.cdc.gov.
National Institutes of Health, National Institute of Diabetes and Digestive and Kidney Diseases: http://www.niddk.nih.gov.

REMEMBER THAT YOU CAN USE LINKS to get from one site to other sites. You can also go to sites through search engines such as Yahoo, Lycos, AltaVista, and Infoseek. But it is essential to be cautious about information provided by sources that are not easily identifiable or well known.

Index

Library of Congress Cataloging-in-Publication Data

Plotnick, Leslie.
  Clinical management of the child and teenager with diabetes / Leslie Plotnick
and Randi Henderson.
      p.   cm. —(The Johns Hopkins Press series in ambulatory pediatric
medicine)
  Includes bibliographical references and index.
  ISBN 0-8018-5908-5 (alk. paper).—ISBN 0-8018-5909-3 (pbk. : alk. paper)
  1. Diabetes in children—Treatment.   I. Henderson, Randi.   II. Title.
III. Series.
  [DNLM: 1. Diabetes Mellitus—therapy.   2. Diabetes Mellitus—in infancy &
childhood.   3. Diabetes Mellitus—in adolescence.   4. Primary Health Care.
WK 815 P729c 1998]
RJ420.D5P58   1998
6128.92'462—dc21
DNLM/DLC
for Library of Congress   98-16878